Jaypee Gold Standard Mini Atlas Series®

PEDIATRIC RADIOLOGY

AF730251

System requirement:

- **Windows XP or above**
- **Power DVD player (Software)**
- **Windows media player 11.0 version or above (Software)**

Accompanying Photo CD ROM is playable only in Computer and not in DVD player.

Kindly wait for few seconds for Photo CD to autorun. If it does not autorun then please do the following:

- Click on my computer
- Click the **CD/DVD drive** and after opening the drive, kindly double click the file **Jaypee**

Radiology is a kindergarten of logical, rational, coherent exploration and balanced learning and not dexterous, adroit, smugness, condescension, superciliousness, disdain or learning egotism cultivated by fake self-centeredness and egoism.

—Hariqbal Singh

Jaypee Gold Standard Mini Atlas Series®

PEDIATRIC RADIOLOGY

Hariqbal Singh MD DMRD
Professor and Head
Department of Radiology
Shrimati Kashibai Navale Medical College, Narhe
Pune 411 041 (Maharashtra), India

JAYPEE BROTHERS MEDICAL PUBLISHERS (P) LTD

New Delhi • St Louis • Panama City • London

Published by

Jitendar P Vij

Jaypee Brothers Medical Publishers (P) Ltd

Corporate Office

4838/24 Ansari Road, Daryaganj, **New Delhi** - 110002, India, Phone: +91-11-43574357
Fax: +91-11-43574314

Registered Office

B-3 EMCA House, 23/23B Ansari Road, Daryaganj, **New Delhi** - 110 002, India
Phones: +91-11-23272143, +91-11-23272703, +91-11-23282021
+91-11-23245672, Rel: +91-11-32558559, Fax: +91-11-23276490, +91-11-23245683
e-mail: jaypee@jaypeebrothers.com, Website: www.jaypeebrothers.com

Offices in India

- **Ahmedabad**, Phone: Rel: +91-79-32988717, e-mail: ahmedabad@jaypeebrothers.com
- **Bengaluru**, Phone: Rel: +91-80-32714073, e-mail: bangalore@jaypeebrothers.com
- **Chennai**, Phone: Rel: +91-44-32972089, e-mail: chennai@jaypeebrothers.com
- **Hyderabad**, Phone: Rel:+91-40-32940929, e-mail: hyderabad@jaypeebrothers.com
- **Kochi**, Phone: +91-484-2395740, e-mail: kochi@jaypeebrothers.com
- **Kolkata**, Phone: +91-33-22276415, e-mail: kolkata@jaypeebrothers.com
- **Lucknow**, Phone: +91-522-3040554, e-mail: lucknow@jaypeebrothers.com
- **Mumbai**, Phone: Rel: +91-22-32926896, e-mail: mumbai@jaypeebrothers.com
- **Nagpur**, Phone: Rel: +91-712-3245220, e-mail: nagpur@jaypeebrothers.com

Overseas Offices

- **North America Office, USA,** Ph: 001-636-6279734
  e-mail: jaypee@jaypeebrothers.com, anjulav@jaypeebrothers.com
- **Central America Office, Panama City, Panama,** Ph: 001-507-317-0160
  e-mail: cservice@jphmedical.com Website: www.jphmedical.com
- **Europe Office, UK,** Ph: +44 (0) 2031708910
  e-mail: dholman@jpmedical.biz; rfurn@jpmedical.biz; pheilbrunn@jpmedical.biz

Jaypee Gold Standard Mini Atlas Series® Pediatric Radiology

First Edition: **2011**

ISBN 978-93-5025-184-3

Typeset at JPBMP typesetting unit

Printed at Ajanta Offset & Packagings Ltd., New Delhi

To

My CT, MR and X-ray technicians
Rahul, Thomas, Raghvendra, Bala,
Premswarup, Mritunjoy, Sudhir,
Deepak, Vinod, Parameshwar and Adi
for their devotion to the field of radiology

CONTRIBUTORS

Abhijit Pawar
Consultant Radiologist
Department of Radiology, Shrimati Kashibai Navale Medical College, Narhe, Pune 411 041 (Maharashtra), India

Amol Nade
Consultant Radiologist
Department of Radiology, Shrimati Kashibai Navale Medical College, Narhe, Pune 411 041 (Maharashtra), India

Amol Sasane
Consultant
Department of Radiology, Shrimati Kashibai Navale Medical College, Narhe, Pune 411 041 (Maharashtra), India

Anand Kamat
Associate Professor
Department of Radiology, Shrimati Kashibai Navale Medical College, Narhe, Pune 411 041 (Maharashtra), India

Ashish Ranade
Lecturer
Department of Orthopedics, Shrimati Kashibai Navale Medical College, Narhe, Pune 411 041 (Maharashtra), India

Parvez Sheik
Consultant Radiologist
Department of Radiology, Shrimati Kashibai Navale Medical College, Narhe, Pune 411 041 (Maharashtra), India

Santosh Konde
Consultant Radiologist
Department of Radiology, Shrimati Kashibai Navale Medical College, Narhe, Pune 411 041 (Maharashtra), India

Sheetal Dhote
Consultant
Department of Radiology, Shrimati Kashibai Navale Medical College, Narhe, Pune 411 041 (Maharashtra), India

Sikandar Shaikh
Consultant
PET-CT Apollo Gleneagles PET-CT Centre
Apollo Health City, Hyderabad, India

Sunila Jaggi MD, DNB, DMRE, DHM
Ex-Associate Professor, Grant Medical College,
Sir JJ Group of Hospitals, Mumbai
Consultant Radiologist, CT Scan and MRI Department,
Bombay Hospital, Mumbai, India

PREFACE

Change is the paramount feature of science and technology, so is true with field of medicine. What is novel today becomes old tomorrow. Therefore, a doctor has to be vigilant and constantly updated with the change. With increase in armaments in the field of imaging, the imaging specialist plays a more decisive role in diagnosis, which is important in treatment.

In this mini atlas more emphasis has been laid on the chapter of 'Brain' which is perplexing, more so after the advent of MRI which has revolutionized the field of pediatrics, particularly neonatal neurology. This has been done at the cost of other chapters which have been truncated, as they are better understood, and at the same instance, prevented this mini atlas on Pediatric Radiology from being voluminous.

This book is meant for the residents, radiologists, pediatricians, general practitioners and other specialists. It is also meant for medical colleges, institutional and departmental libraries and for stand-alone pediatric and imaging establishments.

Hariqbal Singh

ACKNOWLEDGMENTS

I express my gratitude to Professor MN Navale, Founder President, Sinhgad Technical Educational Society and Professor Arvind V Bhore, Dean, Smt Kashibai Navale Medical College for their kind go-ahead in this venture.

I profusely thank the Consultants Prashant Naik, Rahul Ranjan, Rajlaxmi Sharma, Dinesh Pardesi, Mrunalini Shah, Manasi Bhujbal, Anubhav Khandelwal, Sushant Bhadane and Sushil Kachewar for their genuine help in building up this educational entity. I extend appreciation to Perfint Healthcare for providing CT-guided precision biopsy images. I express gratitude to Siemens Ag, Germany for providing MRPET images prior to its commercial launch.

My gratitude to Manjusha Chikale, Nursing Sister, Snehal Nikalje, Anna Bansode and Sachin Babar for their clerical help.

I am thankful and grateful to Almighty and mankind who have allowed me to have this wonderful experience.

CONTENTS

INTRODUCTION

The field of pediatrics comprises of growth, development and wellbeing of the child. It begins when conception is manifested and continues during growth and developmental processes till 21 years of age. However, various institutes consider the upper age for pediatric group from 12 to 21 years.

Pediatrics differs from adult medicine by the obvious body size and maturational changes. The smaller body of an infant or neonate is substantially different physiologically. Congenital defects, genetic variance, and developmental issues are of greater concern to pediatricians than to general physicians, so is true with pediatrics' imaging.

Irradiation *in utero* can lead to developmental abnormalities (8–25 weeks) due to DNA damage and can also lead to malignancy which can be expressed in childhood or during adulthood. Preconception maternal irradiation in therapeutic doses gives rise to defects in 1 out of 10 exposed children. Non-urgent radiological examination should not be done between 8 and 17 weeks of gestation, which is the most sensitive period for organogenesis. Children are 10 times more sensitive for hazards of radiations than adults. Hence, radiography with high kV and low mAs technique is recommended for children to prevent against secondary radiations. Lead or bismuth shields/aprons/protective devices should be used to cover eyes, thyroid, breasts, gonads, whenever possible, particularly in pediatric group, to minimize their exposure to radiations.

CHAPTER
One

Brain

Sunila Jaggi
Abhijit Pawar

CONGENITAL ANOMALIES

Absent Septum Pellucidum

Absence of septum pellucidum can occur in isolation and may be associated with a severely dysmorphic facies, abnormal reflexes and increased tone at birth. When absence of septum pellucidum is associated with hypoplasia of the optic nerve and optic chiasma, it is called septo-optic dysplasia. It is believed to be a mild form of lobar holoprosencephaly (Figure 1.1).

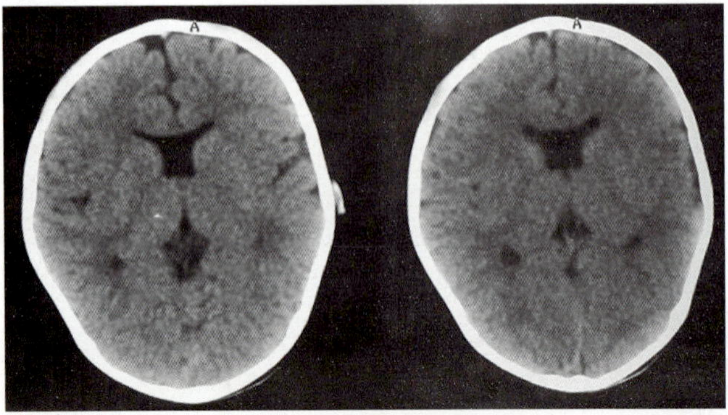

Figure 1.1: Axial CT shows absence of septum pellucidum with resultant appearance of mild form of lobar holoprosencephaly.

Meningocele

Cranial meningocele is herniation of meninges through the skull vault defect. Cranial meningoceles are less frequently seen whereas spinal meningoceles are more common (Figure 1.2).

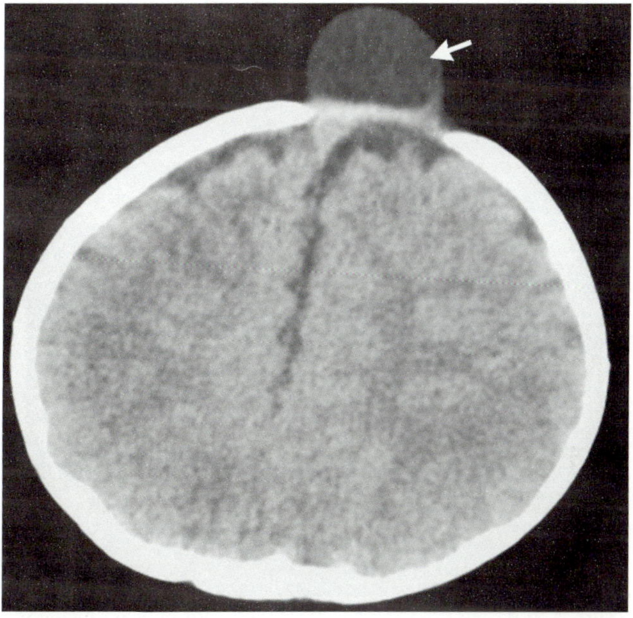

Figure 1.2: Axial CT shows meningocele protruding through the anterior fontanelle.

Aqueduct Stenosis

Aqueduct stenosis is a congenital stenosis of the aqueduct which results in hydrocephalus involving the third and lateral ventricles. While this usually presents in infancy or childhood, in all cases it is necessary to exclude obstructive hydrocephalus due to a local tumor or ependymitis (Figure 1.3).

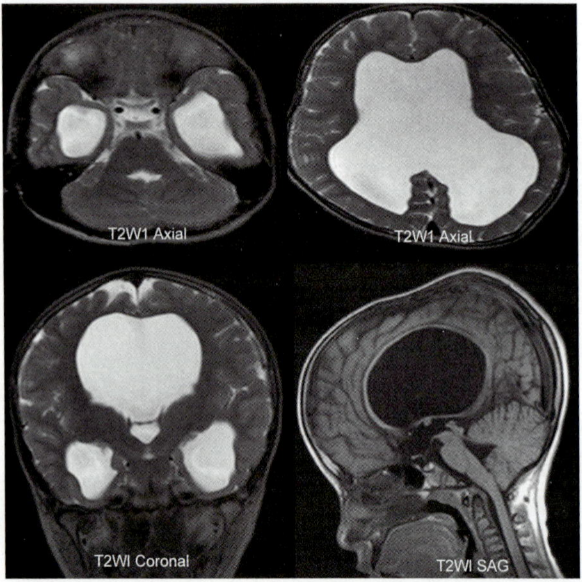

Figure 1.3: 11-year-old female presented with delayed milestones with macrocephaly and giddiness. MRI brain shows dilatation of lateral ventricles and third ventricle. Fourth ventricle appears normal. These findings suggest acqueductal stenosis resulting in moderate to severe hydrocephalus.

Agenesis of Corpus Callosum (ACC) with Interhemispheric Cyst

The association of interhemispheric cysts with ACC is well recognized. Interhemispheric cysts associated with ACC are classified as type 1 cysts, which are diverticula of the lateral or third ventricles and type 2 cysts are loculated and do not appear to communicate with the ventricular system (Figure 1.4).

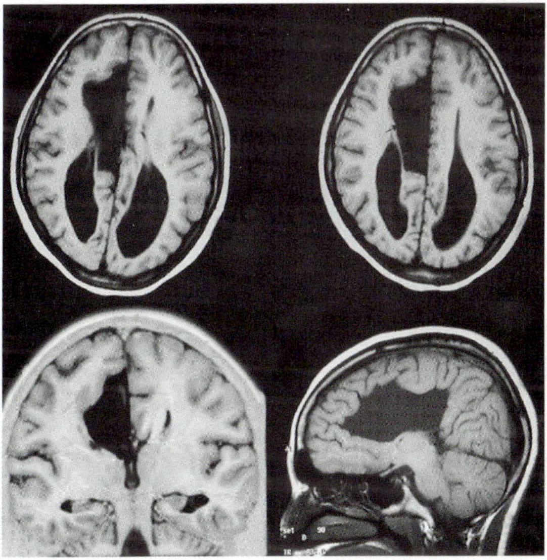

Figure 1.4: MRI shows agenesis of corpus callosum with a right parasagittal interhemispheric cyst (arrow) lined by dysplastic cortex.

Dysgenesis of Corpus Callosum

The corpus callosum is a midline commissure that crosses from one cerebral hemisphere to the other. *Agenesis of corpus callosum* (ACC) is complete or partial absence of the corpus callosum. In ACC, genu is usually present, body and splenium are dysgenic. Signs and symptoms of ACC and other callosal disorders vary, common characteristics include vision impairment, low muscle tone, poor motor coordination, delays in motor milestones, low pain perception, swallowing and chewing difficulties (Figures 1.5A to C).

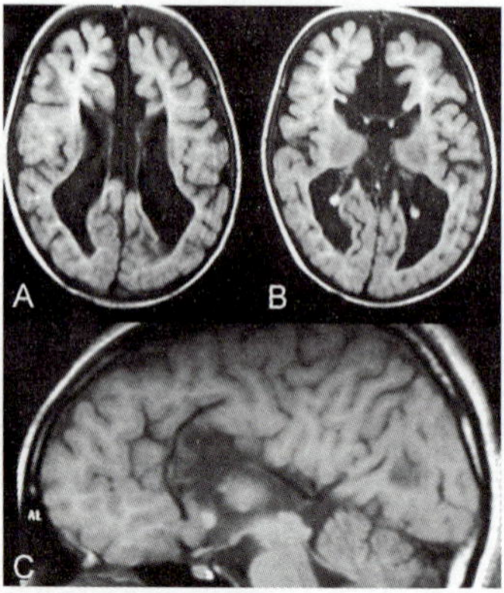

Figures 1.5A to C: A and B—MRI show diagnostic features of parallel nonconverging lateral ventricles with dilated occipital horns (colpocephaly). C—In another case mid-sagittal MR scan shows absence of corpus callosum. Cingulate sulcus is absent and the gyri radiate from a high riding third ventricle.

Schizencephaly

Schizencephaly means split brain. CSF filled cleft extends from the ependymal surface of ventricles to the pia matter. Differential diagnosis of schizencephaly is porencephalic cyst in which the CSF cleft is lined by gliotic white matter, whereas in schizencephaly the cleft is lined by heterotopic gray matter (Figures 1.6A to D).

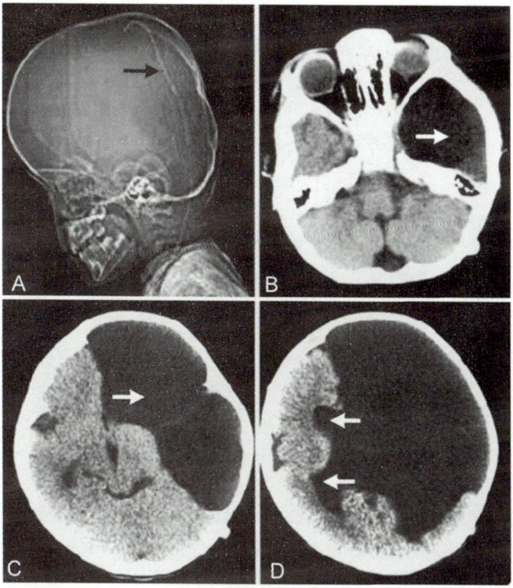

Figures 1.6A to D: A—CT Scanogram shows head with VP shunt. B to D—Shows open lip schizencephaly occupying the left hemicranium.

Open Lip Schizencephaly

Schizencephalies are migrational disorders of brain which are characterized by gray matter lined cleft that extends from the ependymal surface of the brain through the white matter to pia matter (Figure 1.7).

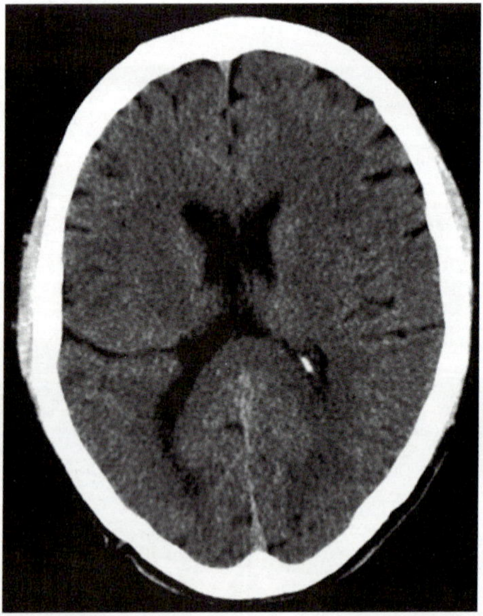

Figure 1.7: Plain CT brain shows a linear CSF density extending from cerebral surface to the ventricle. This CSF density is lined by gray matter.

Lissencephaly

Lissencephaly is the most severe form of the migrational anomaly, in this there is complete or partial absence of sulcation giving appearance of a smooth brain. Lissencephaly children are mentally retarded and have severe seizure disorder with dysmorphic facies (Figure 1.8).

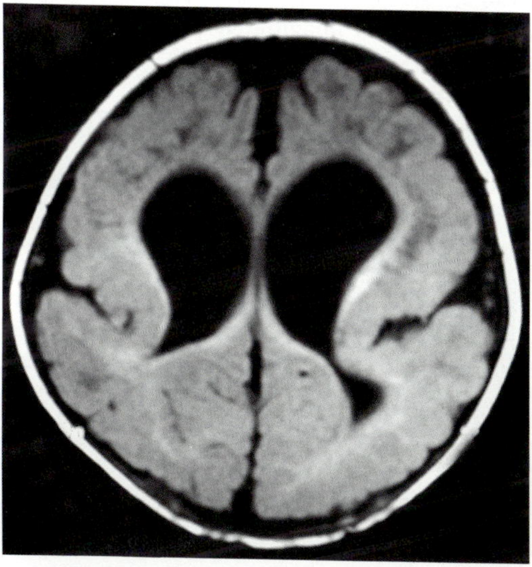

Figure 1.8: MRI shows broad, thick and flat gyri (pachygyria) giving the brain a smooth appearance. There is marked reduction in white matter with dilatation of lateral ventricles. The figure of 8 appearance seen in this image is a typical feature of lissencephaly.

Focal Cortical Dysplasia

Focal cortical dysplasia is a potent epileptic focus in children and leads to disorganization of the normal structure of the cerebral cortex resulting in intractable seizures, however they are amenable to surgical excision. The presence of ectopic neurons and bizarre glial cells, dysmyelination and a reduction in the number of myelinated fibers are likely responsible for the MR imaging characteristics (Figures 1.9A and B).

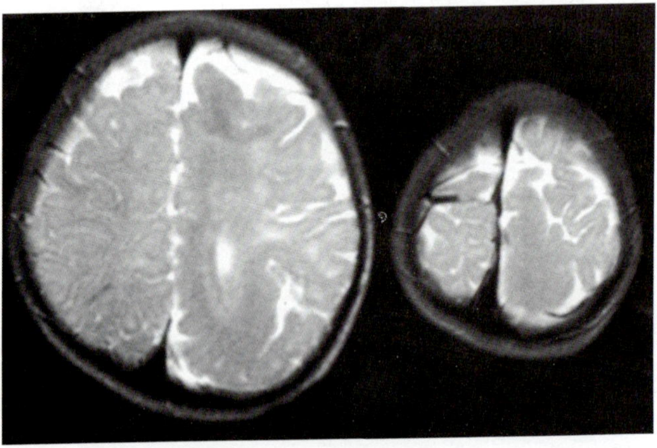

Figure 1.9A: MRI T2WI shows focal cortical enlargement in which sulci and gyri are appreciated. The resultant mass effect on the ipsilateral lateral ventricle and falx, there is dilatation of contralateral lateral ventricle (not seen in the figure).

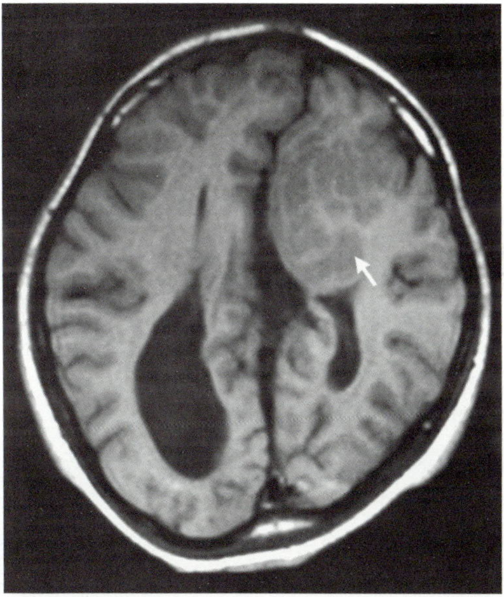

Figure 1.9B: T1-weighted image shows blurring of the gray matter-white matter junction and abnormal signal intensity in the white matter in left cerebral hemisphere.

Arnold-Chiari II Malformation

Chiari malformations (Figures 1.10A to E) are classified as:

Chiari I Malformation—Cerebellar tonsils herniate below foramen magnum > 5 mm, clinical symptoms in form of cranial nerve dysfunctions and/or sensory or motor disturbances in the extremities. Posterior fossa is usually small. This is never associated with meningomyelocele but basilar impression can be present.

Chiari II Malformation—There is dysgenesis of hindbrain associated with caudal displacement of brainstem and fourth ventricle. Cerebellar tonsils and vermis are herniated below foramen magnum. It is associated with lumbar meningomyelocele but never associated with basilar impression. Hydrocephalus is usually present due to dysfunction of aqueduct of Sylvius.

Chiari III Malformation—Characterized by low occipital or high cervical meningomyeloencephalocele.

Chiari IV Malformation—Posterior fossa is small funnel-shaped with cerebellar agenesis and pontine hypoplasia.

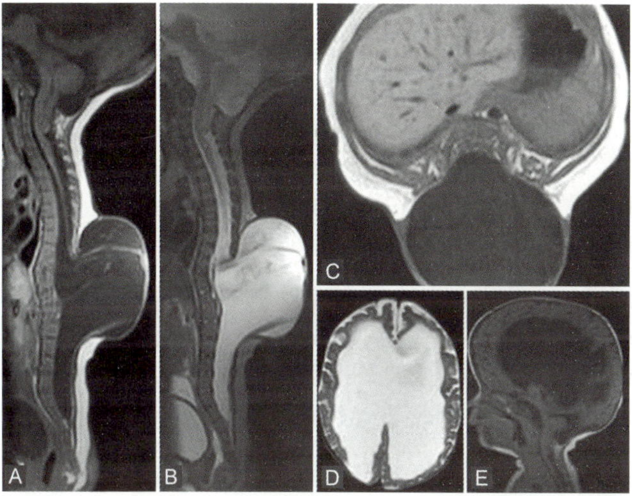

Figures 1.10A to E: One-day-old male neonate with CHIARI II malformation. Presented with swelling on back, no head holding and widely open sutures. MRI on sagittal T1W (A), sagittal T2W (B), axial T1W (C), axial T2W (D) and sagittal T1W (E) images show midline defect in the posterior elements of D9 to L2 vertebrae. A CSF filled sac is seen protruding through this defect beyond the plane of the back. It is not covered with skin. The spinal cord continues into the sac and the neural placode is adherent to the posterior aspect of the sac. Nerve roots are seen traversing through it. Segmentation anomalies are seen in the vertebral bodies at this level. No evidence of lipoma, dermoid, diastematomyelia. Small syrinx is seen in cervical cord. Cerebellar tonsils are peg shaped and low lying. Posterior fossa structures are small. There is severe dilatation of third and both lateral ventricles.

Bilateral Band Heterotopia (Double Cortex)

Heterotopia is presence of normal neural tissue at an abnormal location secondary to arrest of neuronal migration along the radial glial fibers. The abnormally located gray matter is isointense to cortical gray matter in all sequences.

Lamellar or band heterotopia is a homogenous gray matter band between the cerebral cortex and the lateral ventricle surrounded by a zone of white matter (Figure 1.11).

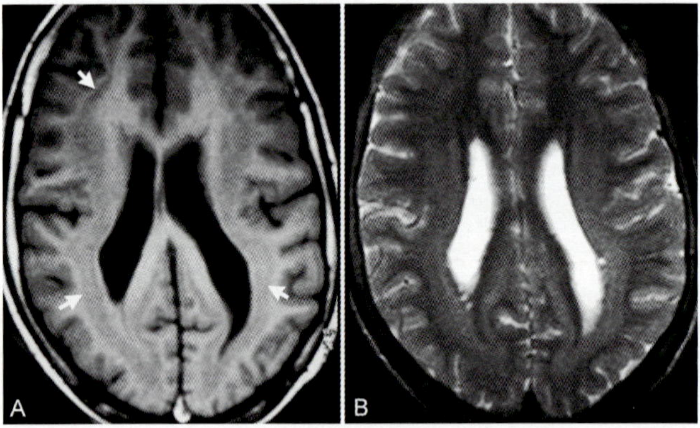

Figure 1.11: MR images show a bilateral band of gray matter (arrows) in the periventricular region similar in intensity to that of gray matter.

Alobar Holoprosencephaly (Arhinencephaly)

Holoprosencephaly is a congenital defect that occurs during the first few weeks of intrauterine life. It is a complex abnormality that results from failure in the diverticulation of the forebrain (prosencephalon). Chromosomal abnormality and trisomy 13 has been associated, maternal infections and paternal toxic exposures have also been implicated. All kinds of holoprosencephalies can be diagnosed by ultrasound. If the sonographic diagnosis is uncertain, MR is diagnostic. Alobar holoprosencephaly is the most severe form of cleavage failure of the forebrain (prosencephalon) before 6 weeks of gestation (Figure 1.12).

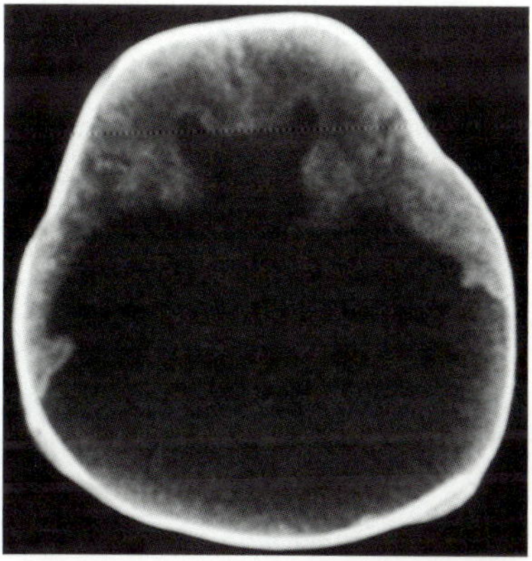

Figure 1.12: Axial CT Scan of a 2 days old child shows a single large ventricular cavity with absence of corpus callosum, falx cerebri and optic tracts.

Perisylvian Syndrome

In perisylvian syndrome, area of the brain called perisylvian region, develops abnormally leading to developmental abnormality and is called polymicrogyria, i.e. abnormal appearance of the cortex with multiple abnormally small convolutions and too few sulci. It is an organization anomaly in which the neurons reach their final destination in the cortex but are distributed abnormally. The thickness of the cortical surface is due to fusion of the adjacent miniature gyri piled upon one another (Figure 1.13).

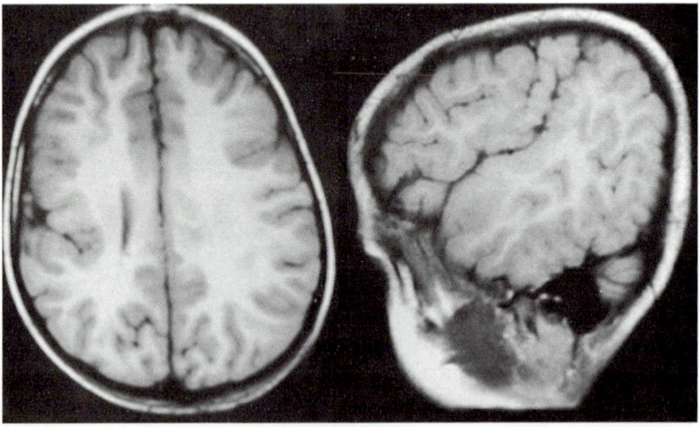

Figure 1.13: MRI shows multiple abnormally small convolutions and too few sulci in an 11-year-old girl who presented with generalized tonic clonic seizures off and on.

Tuberous Sclerosis

Tuberous sclerosis is a rare, multi-system, congenital disorder of autosomal dominant variety that causes benign tumors to grow in the brain. Symptoms may include seizures, developmental delay, behavioral problems, skin abnormalities, lung and kidney diseases. Skin findings include ash leaf-shaped macules, angiofibromas of the face (adenoma sebaceum), congenital shagreen patches and depigmented nevi (Figures 1.14A to C).

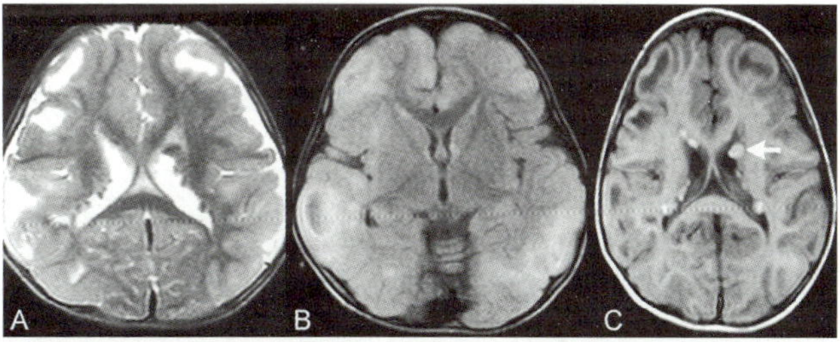

Figures 1.14A to C: Three-year-old female diagnosed as tuberous sclerosis was born of nonconsanguineous marriage presented with delayed language development skills, intermittent hematuria with two episodes of seizures in infancy. She was able to speak only few familiar words.

A—Plain axial T2WI MRI brain.

B—Axial FLAIR MRI demonstrates hyperintense cortical tubers or hamartomas.

C—Post contrast axial MRI images demonstrate enhancement of subependymal tubers.

Benign Enlargement of the Subarachnoid Spaces (BESS)

This is not a congenital anomaly. It has been included in this part only for convenience.

Patients who have BESS have long been suspected of having an increased propensity for subdural hematomas either spontaneously or as a result of accidental injury. Subdural hematomas in infants are often equated with non-accidental trauma (NAT). Caution must be exercised when investigating for NAT based on the sole presence of subdural hematomas, especially in children who are otherwise well and who have BESS (Figures 1.15A and B).

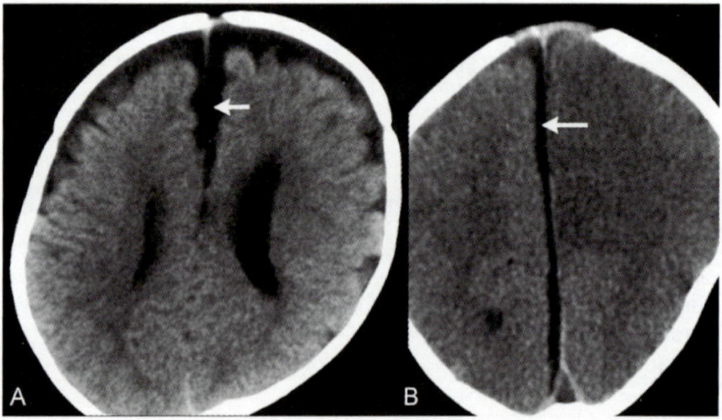

Figures 1.15A and B: CT Brain shows prominent subarachnoid spaces along the interhemispheric fissures.

NEONATAL INSULT

Periventricular Leukomalacia

Periventricular leukomalacia (PVL) is portrayed by death of white matter due to softening of the brain tissue. It can affect fetuses or neonates, premature babies are at the maximum threat, PVL is caused by a lack of oxygen or blood flow to the periventricular area, resulting in loss of brain tissue. Although children with PVL generally have no outward signs or symp-toms of the disorder, they are at threat for epilepsy, motor disorders, delayed mental development, coordination problems, vision and hearing impairments (Figures 1.16A and B).

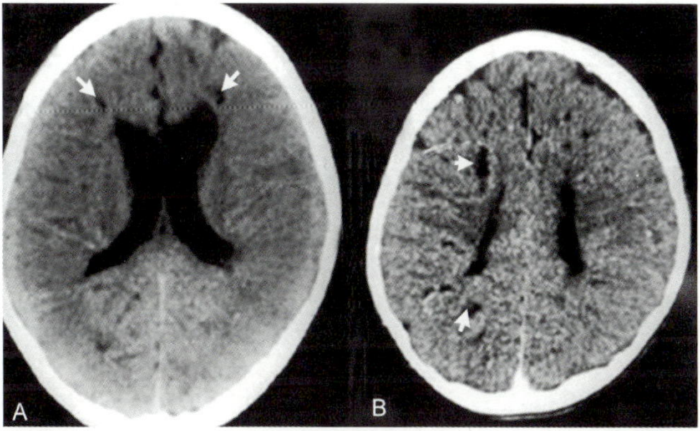

Figures 1.16A and B: PVL in a 4-year-old male child with history of preterm delivery and birth asphyxia. CT shows paucity of periventricular white matter with mild dilatation of the lateral ventricles. The margins of the ventricles are mildly irregular. CSF density lesions (arrows) seen in the periventricular white matter are due to gliosis.

Periventricular Leukomalacia—Chronic

MRI has not been used widely in diagnosis of acute periventricular leukomalacia (PVL), but is extensively used to study chronic PVL. In chronic PVL there is increased T2 signal in the periventricular white matter or gliosis, thinning and loss of volume of periventricular white matter with development of porencephalic cysts, ventriculomegaly and thinning of corpus callosum (Figure 1.17).

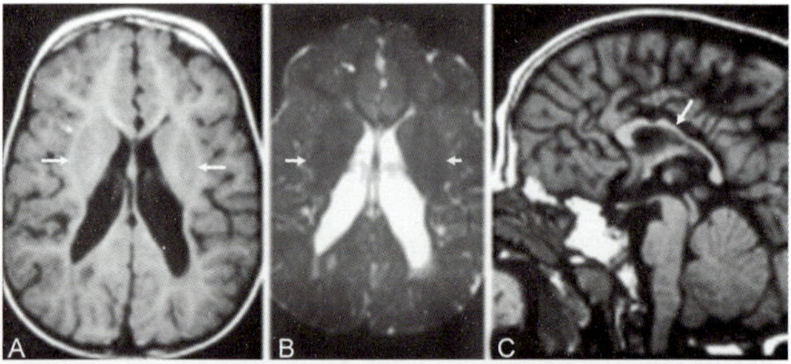

Figure 1.17: T1W (A), T2W (B) axial and T1W sagittal (C) images show that there is paucity of white matter (thin arrow), ventricular dilatation with irregular margins and thinning of the corpus callosum (thick arrow).

Germinal Matrix Hemorrhage—Grade IV

Germinal matrix hemorrhage is a bleeding into the *subependymal germinal matrix* with or without subsequent rupture into the *lateral ventricle*. The caudothalamic groove is a highly *cellular* and highly *vascularized* region in the *brain* from which *cells* migrate out during *brain development*. The germinal matrix is the source of both *neurons* and *glial cells* and is most active between 8 and 28 weeks of *gestation*. It is a fragile portion of the *brain* that may be damaged leading to an *intracranial hemorrhage* known as a *germinal matrix hemorrhage*.

Grade IV refers to intraventricular rupture and hemorrhage into the surrounding white matter (Figures 1.18A and B).

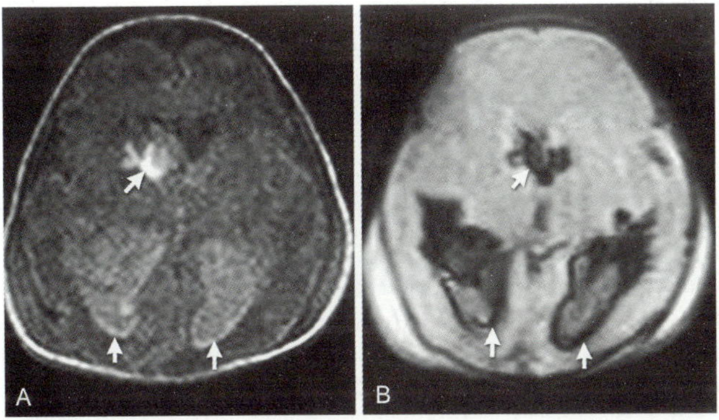

Figures 1.18A and B: T1W axial (A) and GRE axial (B) images reveal hemorrhage in the right germinal matrix with intraventricular extension and associated parenchymal hemorrhage.

Hypoxic Ischemic Encephalopathy

Hypoxic ischemic encephalopathy results from diffuse hypoxic ischemia due to brain insult in the neonate, and MRI is the modality of choice for evaluating the brain injury. In preterm neonates, mild hypotension results in periventricular injury, and severe hypotension in infarction of deep nuclei, brainstem and cerebellum. In full-term neonates mild hypotension results in cortical and subcortical injury and in severe hypotension lateral thalami, hippocampus, brainstem, and cerebellum are affected. Prompt recognition of these imaging findings can help exclude other causes of encephalopathy and affect prognosis (Figures 1.19A to C).

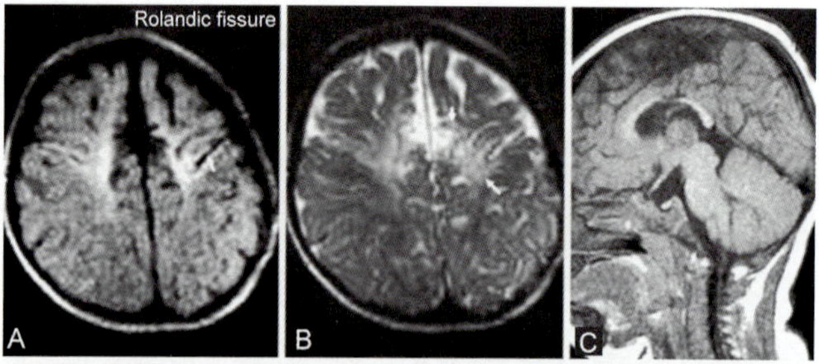

Figures 1.19A to C: 4-month-old child with history of full-term delivery and birth asphyxia shows hypoxic ischemic encephalopathy with involvement of the perirolandic region (Rolandic fissure shown by arrow in A). FLAIR (A), T2WI (B) and sagittal T1WI (C). Hyperintense signal is seen in the perirolandic white matter (arrows) on FLAIR and T2W images. The genu and anterior aspect of the body of the corpus callosum are thin (C).

Global Hypoxia

Global hypoxia is ischemic injury to the brain and results in mortality and severe neurological disability. MRI establishes the diagnosis and plays an important role in treatment and management providing valuable information on long-term prognosis (Figures 1.20A to D).

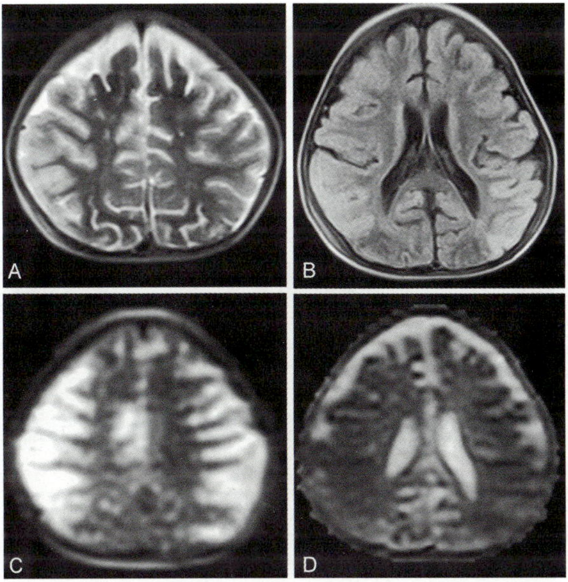

Figures 1.20A to D: Global hypoxic insult in a 2-year-old girl who presented with status epilepticus. T2W (A) and FLAIR (B) images reveal hyperintense signal in the bilateral cortical/subcortical regions with restriction of diffusion on DW (C) and ADC (D) images. This represents cytotoxic edema and is suggestive of prolonged global hypoxia.

Cystic Encephalomalacia

Cystic encephalomalacia is a *cystic* area in the brain *parenchyma* with presence of multiple glial septations. They result from *infarction,* infection or *trauma* and may be *focal* or *diffuse* depending on cause and severity. The presence of glial septations (Figures 1.21A to C) distinguishes *cystic* encephalomalacia from an area of porencephaly and indicates that the injury occurred. On imaging, the cavities and septation are best seen on *MRI* than on *CT. Calcification* may be present and is best seen on *CT.*

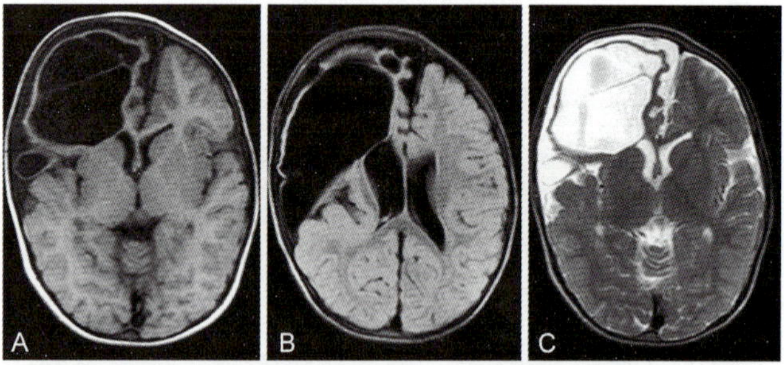

Figures 1.21A to C: Cystic encephalomalacia. CSF intensity lesions with thin walls and few internal septae are seen in the right frontal parenchyma. These lesions appear hypointense on T1W (A) and FLAIR (B) images and hyperintense on T2W images (C). The CSF spaces in this region are prominent. There is loss of white matter with resultant dilatation of the right frontal horn.

INFECTIONS

Meningitis

Infection may be of bacterial, viral, parasitic or fungal in origin and extends to the meninges hematogenously or by direct extension. Initially there is meningeal vascular congestion, edema and micro-focal areas of hemorrhage, followed by involvement of ependymal lining of ventricle and the subpial cortex of brain. Initially CT scan may be normal followed by increased density in the basal cisterns, interhemispheric fissure and choroid plexuses. Postcontrast enhancement in the pachymeninges and leptomeninges and cortical areas is seen (Figures 1.22A to C).

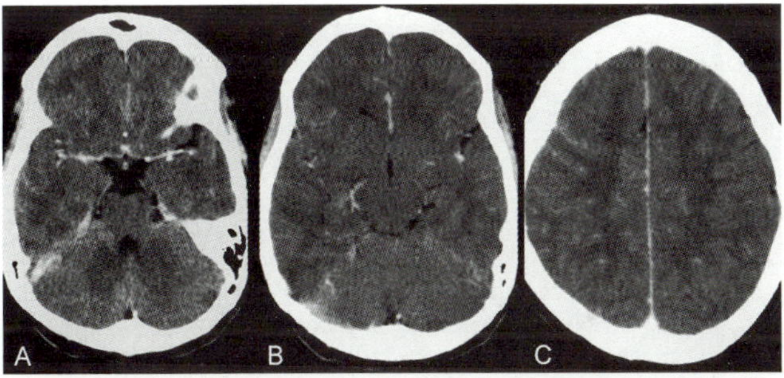

Figures 1.22A to C: 14-year-old female presented with high grade fever, headache, nausea, altered sensorium and positive neck stiffness. Contrast CT brain shows abnormal enhancement along the cerebral sulci, right sylvian fissure and tentorial leaflet suggestive of meningitis.

Cytomegalovirus Infection

Cytomegalovirus (CMV) infection is caused by a species—specific double stranded DNA herpes group virus, which causes an inapparent infection or a "mononucleosis-type" illness in young healthy adults, a chronic disease in older adults and mild to severe congenital infection. An estimated 0.2–2.4% of worldwide live-born infants acquire the virus perinatally. Only 10% of these will demonstrate classic signs of illness at birth. CMV has a particular affinity for the developing germinal matrix in infants but it can infect other organ cells with development of characteristic cytoplasmic or nuclear inclusion bodies. CT scan of the brain shows atrophy, ventricular dilatation and parenchymal calcifications. It can cause widespread parenchymal calcifications in various locations but the subependymal and periventricular region are the most common sites as seen in this case (Figure 1.23).

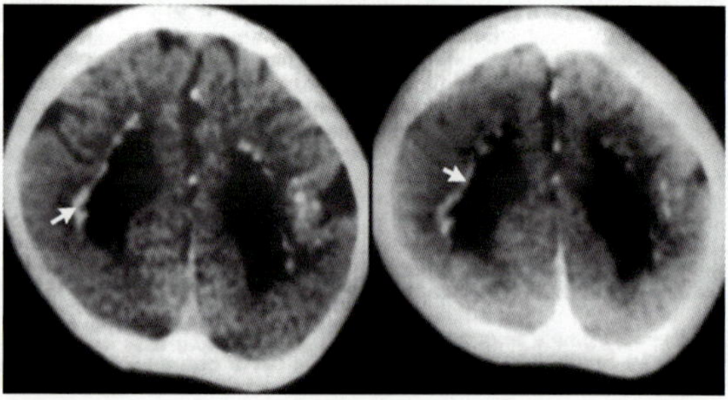

Figure 1.23: A 4-year-old female child presented with delayed milestones and recurrent generalized seizures. Child was found to have microcephaly, optic atrophy, bilateral sensorineural hearing loss, mental retardation and spastic quadriparesis. CT scan of head shows dilated lateral ventricles with non-enhancing subependymal calcifications (arrows) along the lateral walls. Nodular parenchymal calcifications are also noted in the left periventricular region.

Neurocysticercosis

All over the world cysticercosis is the most common parasitic infection of the human central nervous system caused by pork tapeworm *Taenia solium*. Cerebral infection by the larva is usually asymptomatic resulting in a small edematous lesion. The larvae or cysticerci develop into cysts. They mature in 3 months after the ingestion of ova. This stage is often asymptomatic but may result in seizures. The initial small edematous lesion is hyperintense on T2-weighted images. The protoscolex may be indentified as a focal nodule within the cyst and is better demonstrated by MR (Figures 1.24A to D).

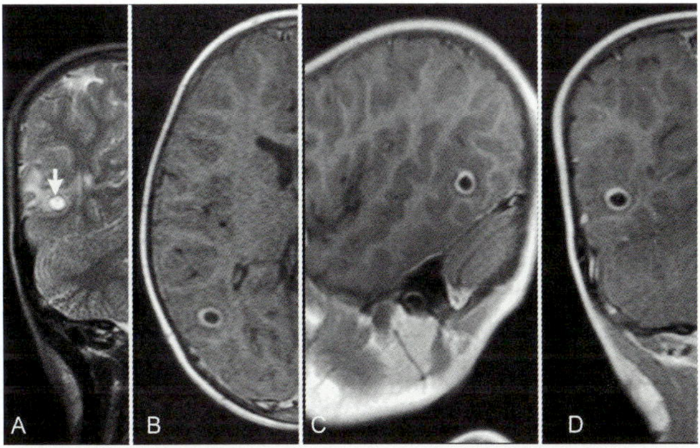

Figures 1.24A to D: In a 6-year-old male, T2W coronal image (A) reveals a small cystic lesion with hypointense rim and eccentric hypointense nodule, surrounding white matter hyperintensity is due to perilesional edema. Postcontrast images B to D reveal smooth peripheral enhancement with mild enhancement of the nodule. This lesion represents cysticercus granuloma and the nodule within it represents the scolex.

Ring Enhancing Lesions

The radiological differential diagnoses of a ring enhancing lesion in the brain would include granuloma, tuberculoma, cysticercus, pyogenic abscess, metastatic disease and a high-grade glioma. Tuberculomas generally have an irregular margin and have significant perilesional edema. Cysticercus granuloma has smooth regular margin and a central scolex. Ring enhancing lesions that can cross corpus callosum are: lymphoma, glioblastoma multiforme and astrocytoma (Figures 1.25A to D).

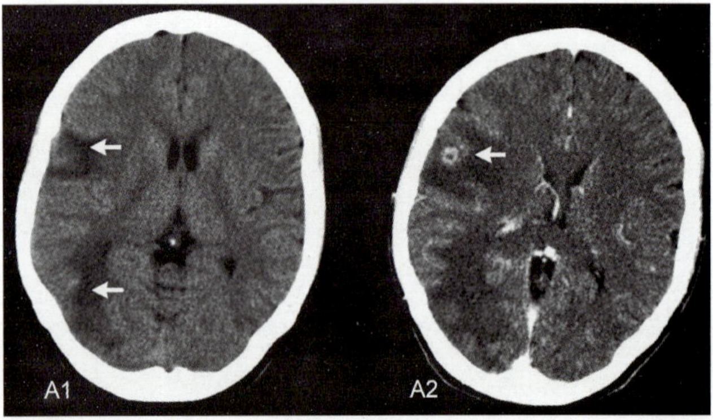

Figure 1.25A: A1—Plain CT Brain shows edema as hypodensities. A2—Contrast CT shows ring enhancing lesion in right fronto-posterior region with surrounding edema.

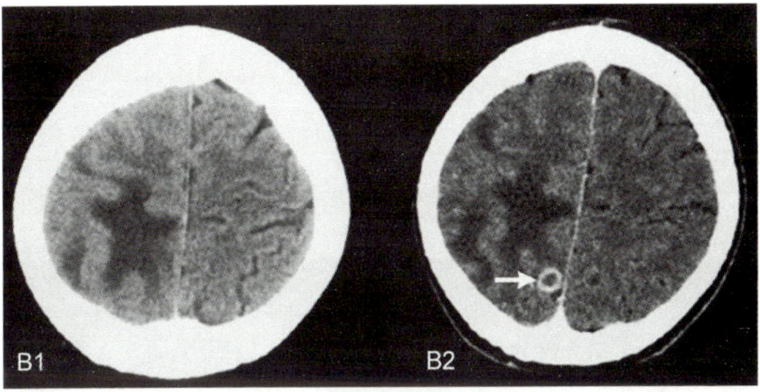

Figure 1.25B: B1—Plain CT Brain showing star shaped hypo-density due to edema. B2—Contrast CT shows ring enhancing lesion in right high parietal region.

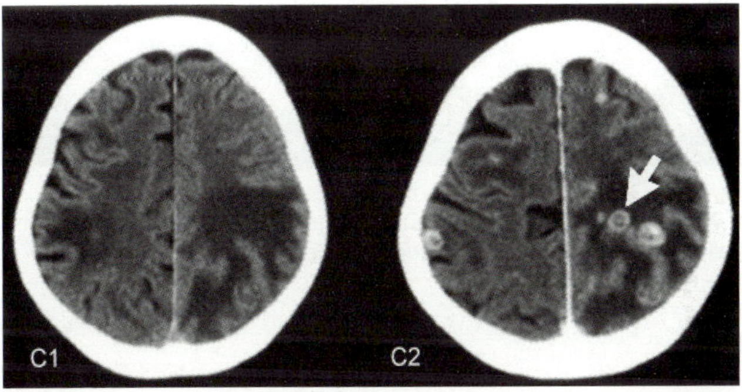

Figure 1.25C: C1—Plain CT Brain shows edema as hypodensities. C2—Contrast CT Brain showing multiple ring enhancing lesions in high parietal region, some of them have a central hyperdense nidus. (neurocysticercosis).

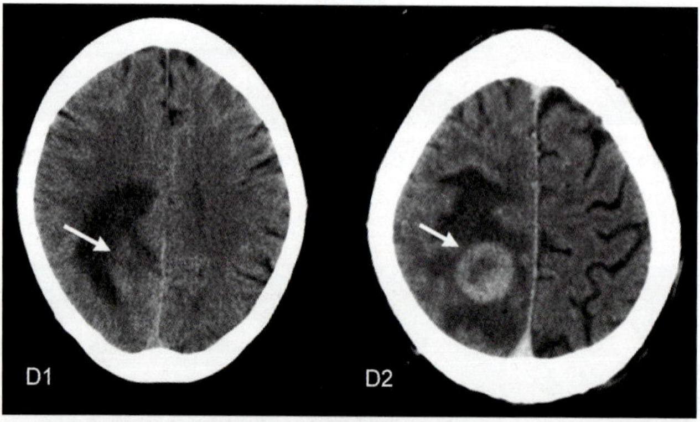

Figure 1.25D: D1—Plain CT Brain showing edema as hypo-density in right high parietal region. D2—Contrast CT Brain showing thick walled enhancing lesion with surrounding edema (Glioma/Metastasis).

Tuberculoma Brain

Common pathological conditions leading to ring enhancing lesions on CT of the brain are granuloma, abscess, some primary brain tumors, resolving hematoma and infarct (Figures 1.26A to D).

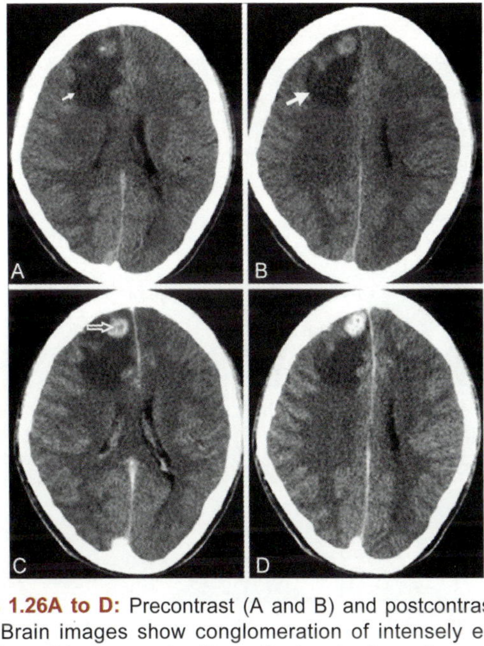

Figures 1.26A to D: Precontrast (A and B) and postcontrast (C and D), CT Brain images show conglomeration of intensely enhancing ring lesions (block arrow) with perilesional edema (arrow) in right frontal lobe.

Tuberculoma 2

Tuberculoma is usually formed by conglomeration of one or several miliary tubercles, which form around the outer sheaths of the small cerebral blood vessels. The center of the conglomeration becomes caseous, inspissated and sometimes liquified. A thick capsule may form around these lesions (Figures 1.27A to E).

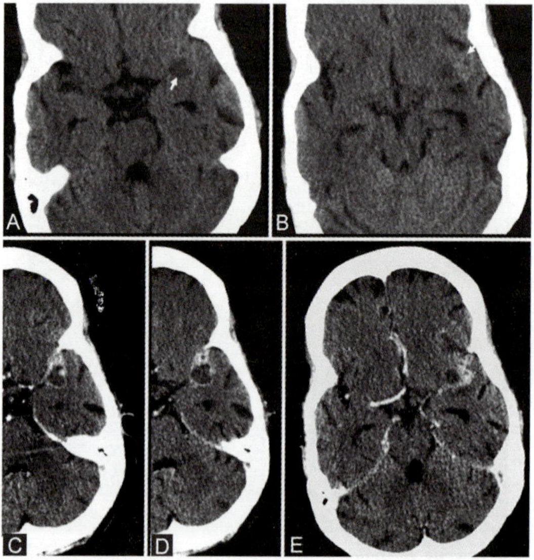

Figures 1.27A to E: A and B—CT images show hypodense areas in the left anterior temporal region. C, D and E—Postcontrast images show multiple ring enhancing tuberculoma. Adjacent leptomeningeal enhancement is also seen.

Calcified Tuberculoma

Follow-up CT in a known case of tuberculoma generally ends up with a calcified focus. However, an initial scan with focal calcification poses a diagnostic dilemma (Figures 1.28A to C).

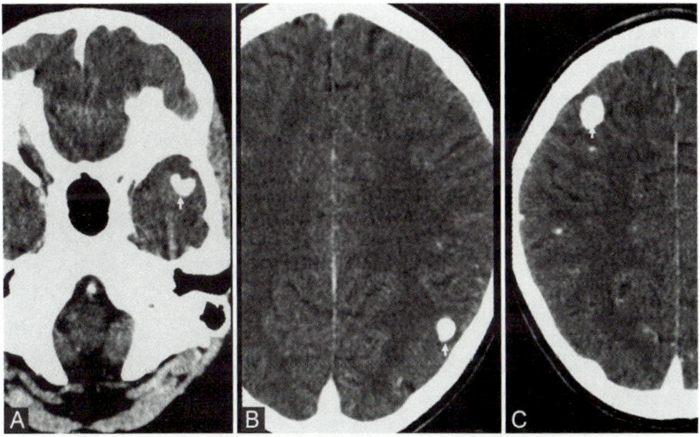

Figures 1.28A to C: A known case of tuberculoma on completion of antitubercular therapy. CT scan shows multiple calcified nodules.

LEUKODYSTROPHY

Adrenoleukodystrophy

X-linked adrenoleukodystrophy (ALD) is a peroxisomal disorder that affects the white matter of the CNS, adrenal cortex and testes. The genetic defect liable for X-linked ALD is located in Xq28, the terminal segment of the long arm of the X chromosome. In X-linked ALD there is a strong association between the presence of contrast enhancement on the T1-weighted MR images and disease progression revealed by clinical evaluation and MR imaging (Figures 1.29A and B).

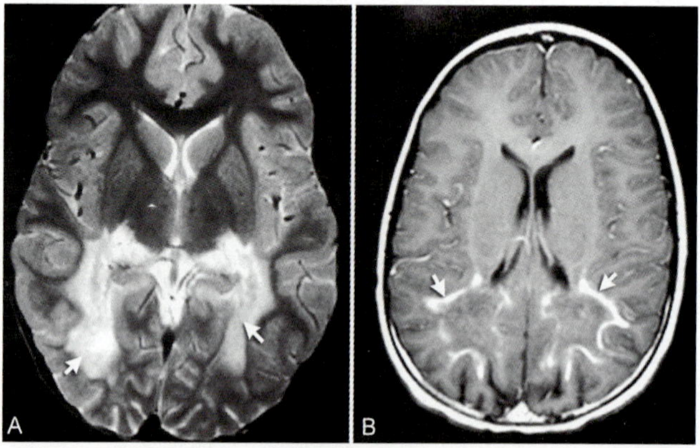

Figures 1.29A and B: X-linked adrenoleukodystrophy. Symmetrical hyperintense signal is seen in the bilateral peritrigonal white matter on T2W image (A). The subcortical white matter is spared. There is no mass effect. On postcontrast T1W image (B) bilateral peripheral enhancement of the lesion is noted, representing active demyelination. These findings are suggestive of X-linked adrenoleukodystrophy.

Metachromatic Leukodystrophy

Metachromatic leukodystrophy (MLD) is a lysosomal storage disease. There is impairment of growth or development of the myelin sheath. All forms of the disease involve a progressive worsening of motor and neurocognitive function. As the word implies, the presence of white matter abnormalities on brain images is characteristic (Figure 1.30).

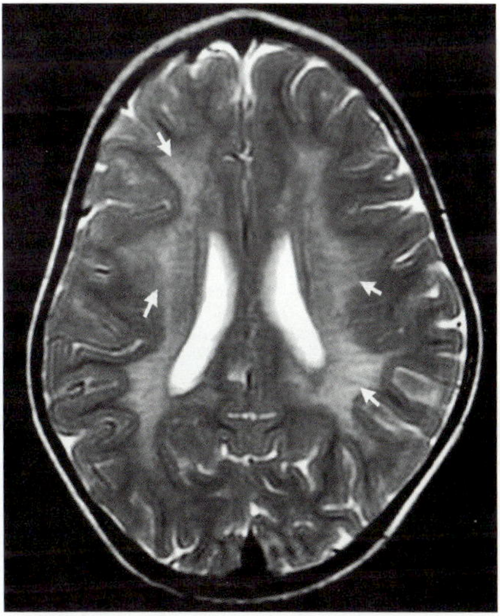

Figure 1.30: T2W image reveals diffuse hyperintense signal (arrows) in the white matter extending to corona radiata on both sides. There is sparing of the subcortical white matter. There is no evidence of mass effect.

Mucopolysaccharidoses

Diagnosis of mucopolysaccharidoses is made by the characteristic urinary mucopolysaccharides combined with the clinical picture. On imaging, the brain shows atrophy, hydrocephalus and sometimes megalocephaly. On MR, multiple dilated perivascular spaces are seen on the T2 weighted axial image (Figures 1.31A and B).

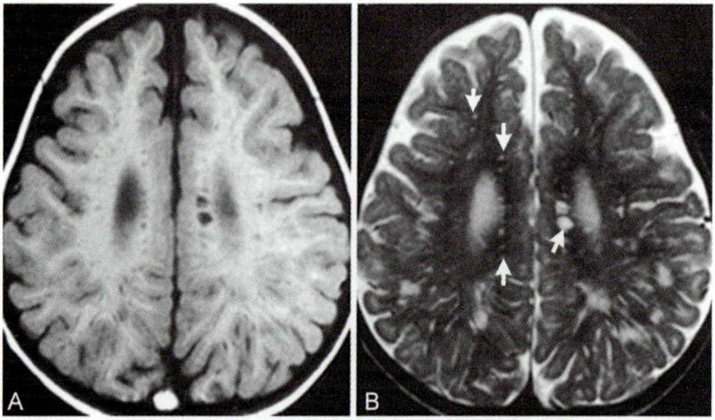

Figures 1.31A and B: MRI in mucopolysaccharidosis shows dilated Virchow-Robin spaces (arrows) which are seen bilateral in the periventricular white matter.

Alexander Disease

Alexander disease is a nonfamilial leukoencephalopathy that presents with frontal preponderance of white matter abnormalities and macrocephaly. MR imaging is known for its high sensitivity and specificity in identifying white matter disorders. Failure of normal myelination is most likely responsible for abnormal white matter signal on MR images (Figure 1.32).

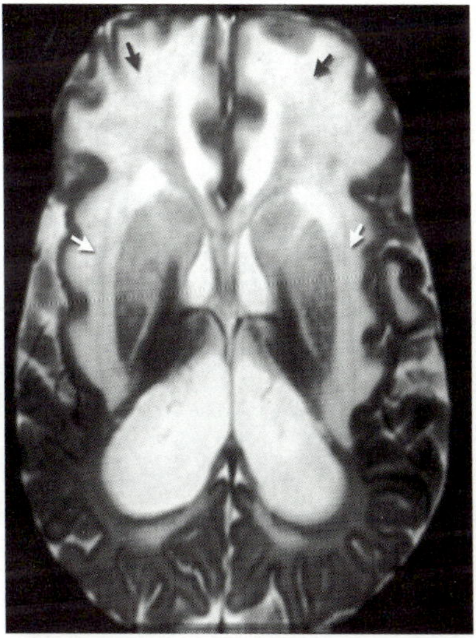

Figure 1.32: T2W image reveals extensive hyperintense signal suggestive of demyelination in the bilateral frontal white matter (black arrows) and external capsules (white arrows).

TUMORS

Epidermoid and Arachnoid Cyst

Arachnoid cyst is a fluid-filled cyst lined with arachnoid membrane. Epidermoid is a benign tumor formed by inclusion of epidermal elements, especially at the time of closure of the neural groove, and located in the skull, meninges or brain. Diffusion-weighted imaging can be used to distinguish epidermoid cyst from arachnoid cyst in the intracranial compartment. On diffusion-weighted image, epidermoid appears bright and arachnoid cyst appears dark. Both conditions may occur simultaneously in the same patient (Figures 1.33A to D).

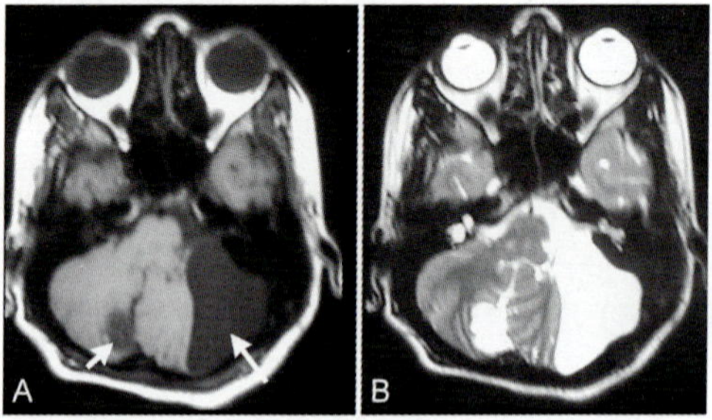

Figures 1.33A and B: Two lesions are seen in the cerebellum. Both appear hypointense on T1W image (A) and hyperintense on T2W image (B).

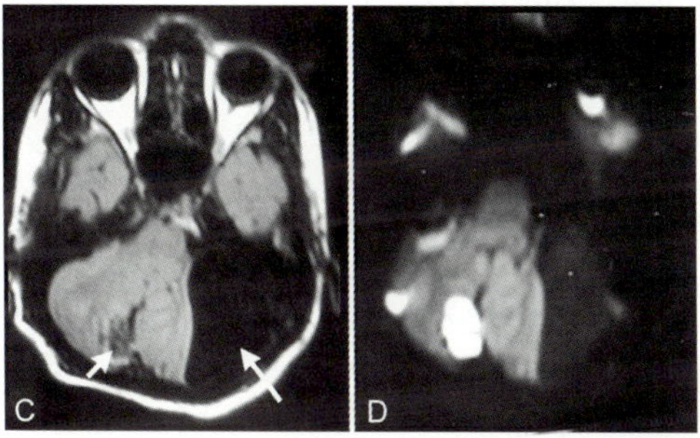

Figures 1.33C and D: On FLAIR (C) image the lesion in the right paramedian region (short arrow) shows mild internal inhomogeneity and the left lesion (long arrow) shows homogeneous suppression of signal. On diffusion-weighted image (D) the smaller lesion on right side appears bright and the lesion on left appears dark. These findings are suggestive of an epidermoid cyst on right side and an arachnoid cyst on left side.

Pineal Epidermoid

On imaging, the characteristic appearance of an epidermoid tumor is that of a smoothly contoured CSF like mass. On CT, it is seen as a non-enhancing hypodense extra-axial mass. MR imaging is the preferred modality to distinguish epidermoid tumor from arachnoid cysts. FLAIR and diffusion-weighted (DW) are the preferred sequences for differentiating them. These sequences confirm the solid nature of epidermoid tumour. Unlike arachnoid cysts which appear isointense to CSF on FLAIR images, the epidermoid appear heterogeneous and relatively higher in signal than CSF. On DW images, epidermoids typically appear hyperintense due to restricted diffusion. The majority of the epidermoids do not show any postcontrast enhancement (Figures 1.34A to D).

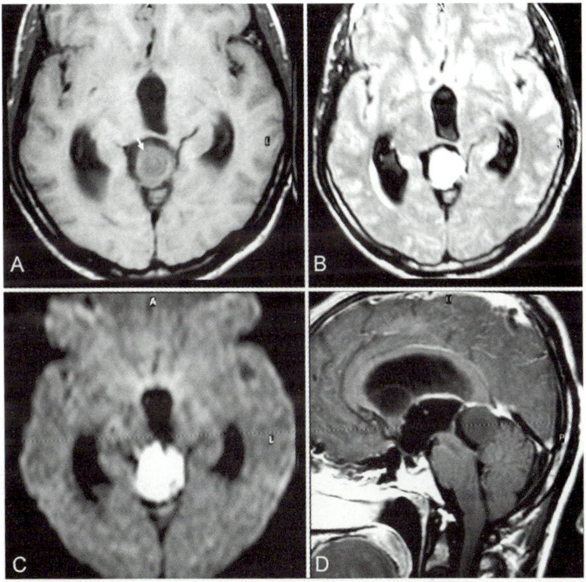

Figures 1.34A to D: A well defined extra-axial lesion is seen in the quadrigeminal plate cistern. It is hypointense on T1W (A), hyperintense on FLAIR (B) and diffusion (C) images and does not enhance on contrast image (D). It compresses the posterior third ventricle leading to moderate hydrocephalous. The extra axial location and MRI finding are suggestive of pineal epidermoid.

Hypothalamic Hamartoma

Hypothalamic hamartoma is a congenital malformation, composed of normal neuronal tissue located between mammillary bodies and tuber cinereum of hypothalamus. It may be sessile or pedunculated, few millimeters to few centimeters in diameter, without calcification or hemorrhage. CT picks up only larger lesions seen as rounded, well defined, homogenous, isodense, non-enhancing lesion. On T1WI, the hamartoma is isointense to gray matter and T2WI is iso- to slightly hyperintense and shows no enhancement (Figures 1.35A to C).

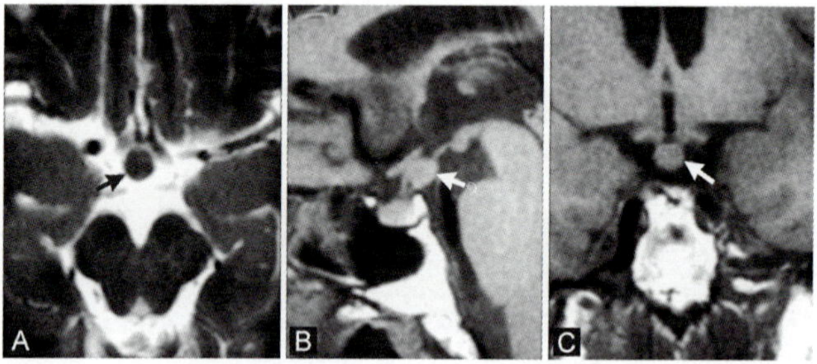

Figures 1.35A to C: T2 Axial (A), Sagittal (B) and Coronal T1W (C) images reveal a well defined oval lesion in between the infundibulum and the mammillary bodies. It is isointense to gray matter on T1 and T2 W images.These lesions do not calcify or enhance.

Chiasmatic/Hypothalamic Astrocytoma

Astrocytomas of the optic chiasma and optic nerve represent approximately 3–5% of brain tumors in children and are usually seen between two to nine years of age. Hypothalamic astrocytomas are usually pilocytic. MRI is the imaging modality of choice. It allows assessment of degree of optic pathway involvement. Chiasmatic gliomas can be hard to distinguish from hypothalamic gliomas when the tumors are big because it is not clear whether the optic chiasma glioma is extending posteriorly into the hypothalamus or whether the hypothalamic glioma is involving the optic chiasma. This is also not necessary because both chiasmatic and the hypothalamic astrocytomas are treated in the same way (Figures 1.36A to C).

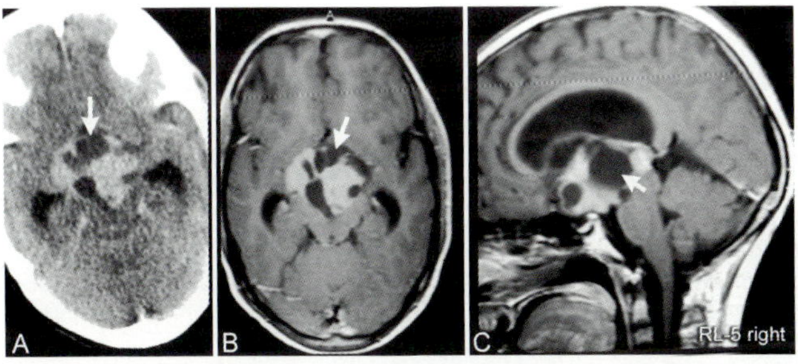

Figures 1.36A to C: Large lobulated heterogeneous lesion is seen in the suprasellar region. On postcontrast CT scan (A) it has a solid enhancing component and a cystic component. Postcontrast axial T1W (B) and sagittal T1W (C) images reveal an enhancing lesion with cystic component in the suprasellar region with involvement of the hypothalamus, optic chiasma and optic nerves. It has compressed the third ventricle and there is mild dilatation of the lateral ventricles.

Craniopharyngioma

Craniopharyngioma arises from remnants of cranio-pharyngeal duct. 50% of suprasellar tumors in children are craniopharyngioma with first peak at 10 to 14 years and second peak at 4th to 6th decade (Figures 1.37A to C).

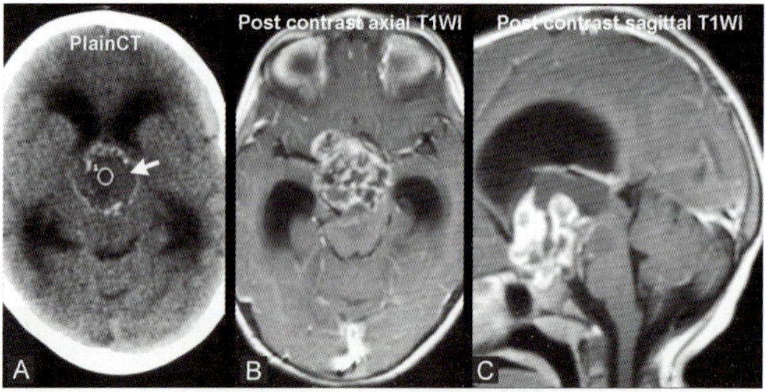

Figures 1.37A to C: A—Plain axial CT reveals a well defined iso- to hypo-dense lesion with a peripheral rim of calcification in the sellar-suprasellar region. Postcontrast axial T1W (B) and sagittal (C) images in a different patient reveal a well defined heterogeneously enhancing lesion in the sellar and suprasellar region with enhancing solid component and non-enhancing cystic component. The ventricular dilatation in both cases is due to compression of third ventricle.

Pontine Glioma

Pontine gliomas range from low grade tumors which necessitate little treatment to those that are rapidly fatal despite aggressive therapy. Prognosis and treatment depend upon the histology and location within the brainstem. Approximately 80 percent of pediatric pontine gliomas arise within the pons, while the remaining 20 percent arise in the medulla, midbrain or cervicomedullary junction. Histologically, these tumors are either anaplastic astrocytomas or glioblastoma multiforme (Figures 1.38A to C).

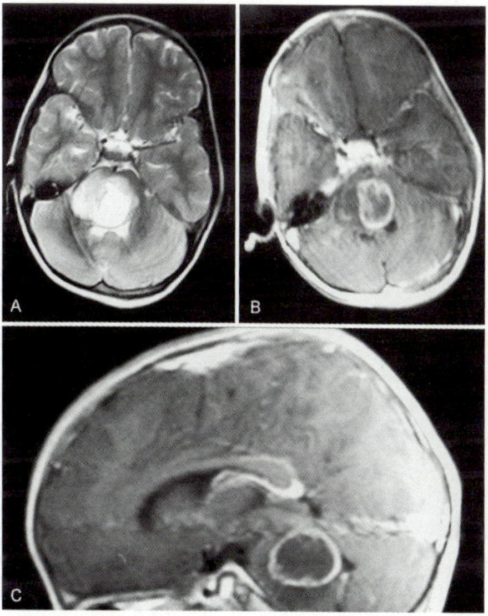

Figures 1.38A to C: Axial T2W image (A), postcontrast axial (B) and sagittal (C) images reveal a large heterogeneous lesion in the pons. A part of it shows peripheral enhancement and rest of it shows mild patchy enhancement. There is mild peri-lesional edema. The fourth ventricle is compressed.

Bilateral Acoustic Schwannomas

Acoustic schwannomas originate from the schwann cells of nerves. It selectively involves the VIII cranial nerve as compared to other cranial nerves. They show focal growth and may have mass effect on adjacent structures and do not undergo malignant degeneration. On CT scans they appear isodense with brain parenchyma but show bright enhancement on contrast scans. On MR T1W images the lesions are hypointense to isointense with brain parenchyma. On T2W images, acoustic schwannomas are hyperintense. Widening of internal acoustic meatus may be seen (Figures 1.39A and B).

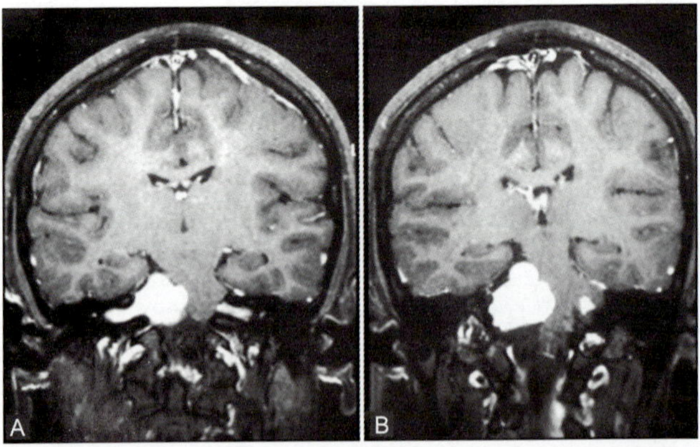

Figures 1.39A and B: Postcontrast coronal T1W images show intensely enhancing bilateral cerebellopontine angle cistern lesions. The right is larger than the left. The lesion on the right side shows extension into the internal auditory meatus.

Cystic Cerebellar Astrocytoma

Cystic cerebellar astrocytoma or pilocytic astrocytoma occurs in children and young adults up to 20 years of age. Cystic astrocytoma usually arises in the cerebellum. It may arise in the brainstem, hypothalamic region or optic chiasma, but may occur in any area where astrocytes are present. They are usually slow growing but invasive, the neoplasms are associated with the formation of a single or multiple cysts and can become very large. It is considered a benign tumor. It is often cystic, if solid, it is well-circumscribed. It characteristically enhances with contrast.

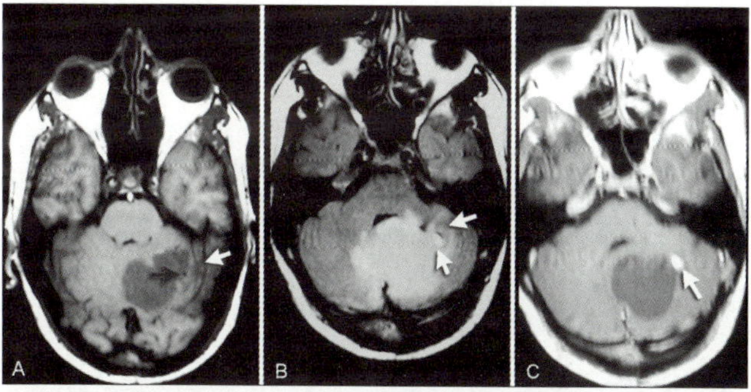

Figures 1.40A to C: A—Axial T1W image shows a cystic lesion in the left cerebellar hemisphere with a small isointense mural nodule (white arrow). Small flow voids is seen due to high velocity blood flow in the vessels that supply the nidus (black arrow). B—The cyst is hyperintense on T2W image and the mural nodule remains isointense (white arrow). C—Postcontrast T1W axial image reveals intense enhancement of the mural nodule (white arrow) in cystic of cystic cerebellar astrocytoma.

Medulloblastoma

Medulloblastoma is a primitive neuroectodermal tumor (PNET) of children and consists of 15% of the malignant brain tumors and 35% posterior fossa tumors of childhood. It arises from external granular cell of the cerebellar folia. 85% of medulloblastoma arise in the posterior fossa, between 5 and 15 years of age. They appear well circumscribed but are frequently invasive. 80% tumors, arise in the roof of the fourth ventricle in the region of vermis and velum in the midline. They pack up to a large extent the fourth ventricle resulting in obstructive hydrocephalus.

On CT the medulloblastoma is isodense to hypodense. Few show calcification (20%). On MRI the lesion is isointense or hypointense on T1WI and isointense to hypointense on T2WI. T2 signal is heterogeneous if calcification, cystic change, hemorrhage or necrosis is present . Tumor shows enhancement both on CT and MRI (Figures 1.41 and 1.42).

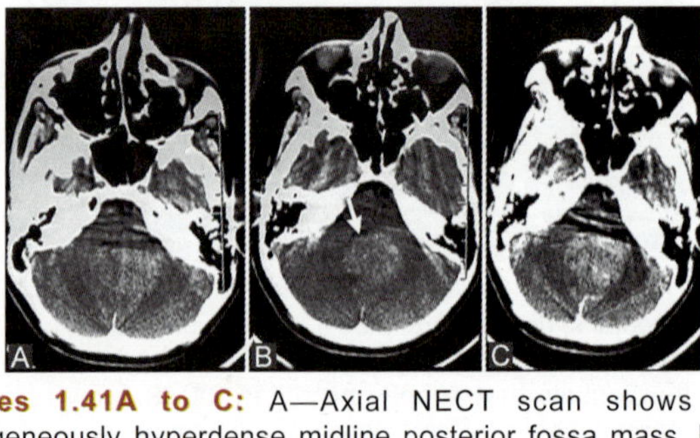

Figures 1.41A to C: A—Axial NECT scan shows round homogeneously hyperdense midline posterior fossa mass. B—The fourth ventricle is markedly compressed (arrow) and mildly displaced anteriorly. B and C—CECT scan shows moderate enhancement. Other sections show dilatation of lateral ventricles.

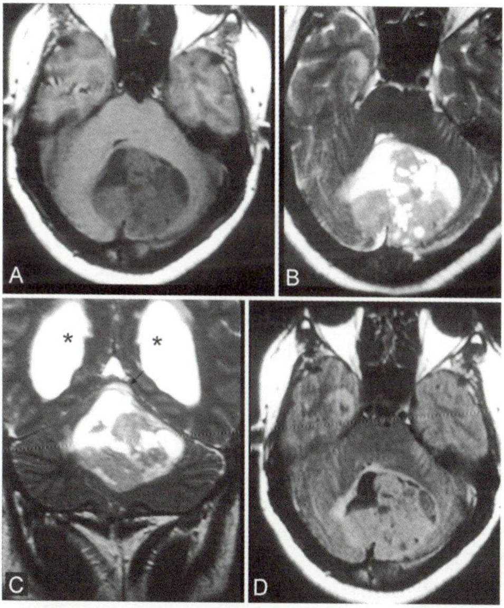

Figures 1.42A to D: Well defined heterogeneous lesion with solid and cystic components is seen in the posterior fossa involving the vermis. The solid component is isointense on T1W image (A), iso- to mildly hyper-intense on T2W image (B) and reveals moderate enhancement on postcontrast image (D). The cystic component is hypointense on T1W image and hyperintense on T2W images. It compresses the fourth ventricle (arrow) causing moderate dilatation (*) of the lateral ventricles (C).

Neurofibromatosis Type 2 (NF2)

Neurofibromatosis is inherited nerve sheath disorder with two distinct types, neurofibromatosis type 1 (NF1) and neurofibromatosis type 2 (NF2). NF1 is von Recklinghausen disease. It is 10 times more common than NF2. NF1 has prominent superficial tumors (neurofibromas), macular hyper pigmentation (café-au-lait spots) and CNS abnormalities that include true neoplasms, usually optic nerve gliomas, dysplastic and hamartomatous lesions. Multifocal increased signal intensiy is seen on T2WI in brainstem, cerebellar white matter, dentate nucleus, basal ganglia, periventricular white matter, optic nerve and optic pathways. These hyperintensities represent either abnormal myelination or hamartomatous change. The presence of bilateral optic nerve gliomas is considered diagnostic for NF1 (Figures 1.43 and 1.44).

NH2 commonly affects the acoustic nerve, trigeminal nerve being next in frequency. They are predisposed to intracranial or intraspinal meningiomas.

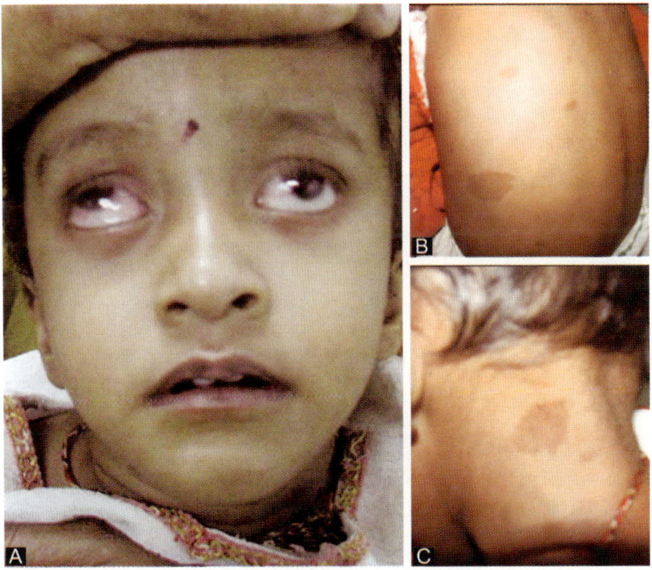

Figures 1.43A to C: (A) Photograph of patient showing squint; (B and C) showing café-au-lait spots.

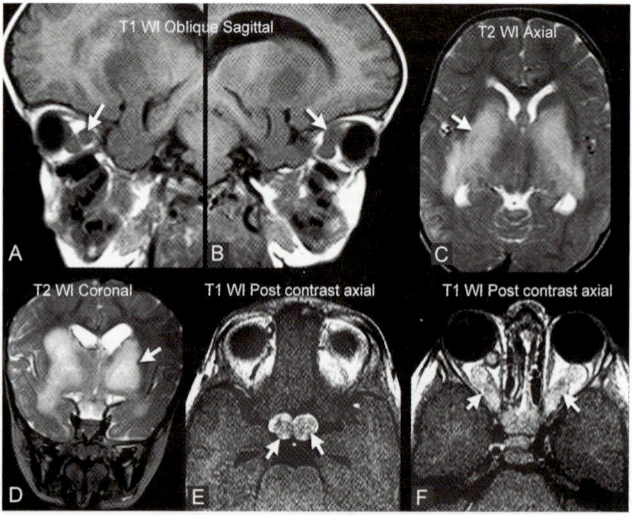

Figure 1.44A to F: Oblique sagittal T1W images show (A) right and (B) left tortuous and enlarged optic nerves (arrow). T2WI (C) axial and (D) coronal images show abnormal hyperintense signal in both gangliocapsular region and along optic tracts. Axial postcontrast T1WI showing (E) enlarged enhancing optic chiasma and (F) bilateral tortuous and enlarged enhancing optic nerves.

Orbital Rhabdomyosarcoma

Orbital rhabdomyosarcoma is the commonest primary orbital malignancy of childhood. Rhabdomyosarcomas are the most common soft tissue sarcoma in childhood accounting for approximately 8% of all childhood malignancy. Ten percent of pediatric rhabdomyosarcomas occur in the orbit. Most series report an average age of about 7–8 years at presentation. The lesions typically present with unilateral proptosis (Figures 1.45A to F).

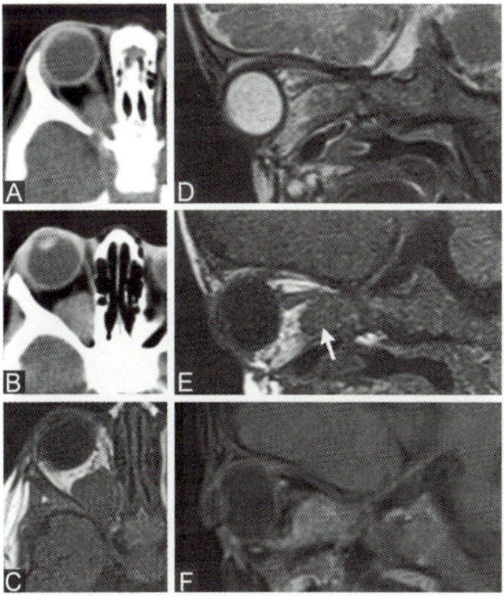

Figures 1.45A to F: Well defined intraconal lesion is seen in the right retro-orbital space closely abutting the inferior rectus muscle and the optic nerve. The optic nerve is mildly displaced superiorly. It appears hypodense on CT scan (A and B), hypointense on T1W (C and E) and iso- to mildly hypo-intense on T2W (D) image. On postcontrast image (F) it shows moderate homogeneous enhancement.

CHAPTER
Two

Vertebral Column

Abhijit Pawar
Santosh Konde

DIASTEMATOMYELIA

Diastematomyelia is a form of spinal dysraphism in which the spinal cord is split into two hemicords each covered by pia mater. Each hemicord contains a central canal and has both dorsal and ventral horns. In most of the cases the hemicords are enclosed by one subarachnoid space and dural sac. There may be a bony spur/fibrous band in between the hemicords. It is common in lower thoracic and lumbar spine. Syrinx may be associated. Other vertebral anomalies may be associated (Figures 2.1A to E).

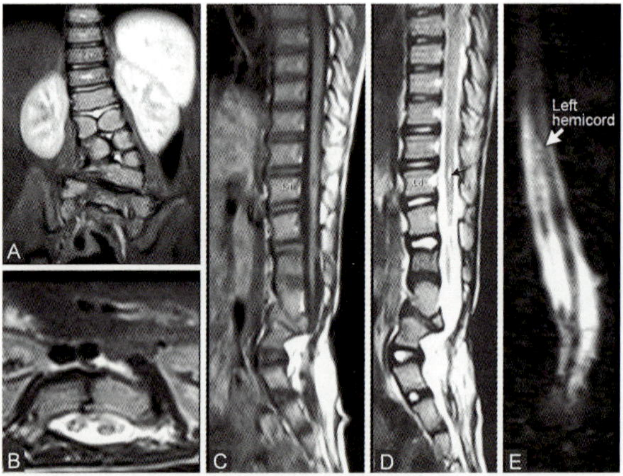

Figures 2.1A to E: Coronal T2 (A), Axial T2W (B), Sagittal T1W (C), Sagittal T2W (D), MR myelography (E) images. Segmentation anomalies are seen in the lumbar vertebrae in the form of cleft vertebrae at L2 and L3 levels and hemivertebra at L4 level (A). The cord is tethered at L4–5 level (C). There is vertical splitting of the cord from L1 to L4 and two hemicords with separate central canals are seen in this region (B). Small syrinx is seen in the cord at D12–L1 level (arrow). The splitting of cord is better demonstrated in the myelography image (E).

MULTIPLE CONGENITAL SPINAL DEFORMITIES

Congenital osseous *anomalies* of the *cervical spine* may perhaps indicate congenital malformations of cardiac and renal systems. However, most *anomalies* are innocuous and may go unnoticed throughout life. Majority of the individuals with congenital *anomalies* of the *cervical spine* are asymptomatic or have only mild constraint of neck movement. If symptoms develop, they are usually due to cervical instability or degenerative osteoarthrosis (Figures 2.2A to C).

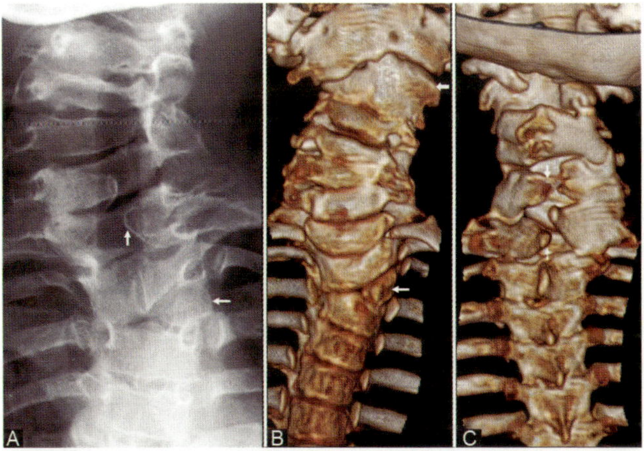

Figures 2.2A to C: Seven-year-old female child presented with mild torticolis. Cervical spine shows fusion of C2, C3 body (arrow) and left lateral elements. Multiple defects of posterior elements of lower cervical vertebrae are seen. Hemivertebra seen at D3 level with scoliosis deformity in upper dorsal spine.

PNEUMORRHACHIS

Pneumorrhachis is existence of air within the spinal epidural space. It is usually iatrogenic or associated with trauma and is rare in asthma. This occurs due to lack of fascial wall between the posterior mediastinum and the retropharyngeal and epidural spaces; as a result, air can diffuse freely to the epidural space and create pneumorrhachis. It is usually asymptomatic (Figures 2.3A to C).

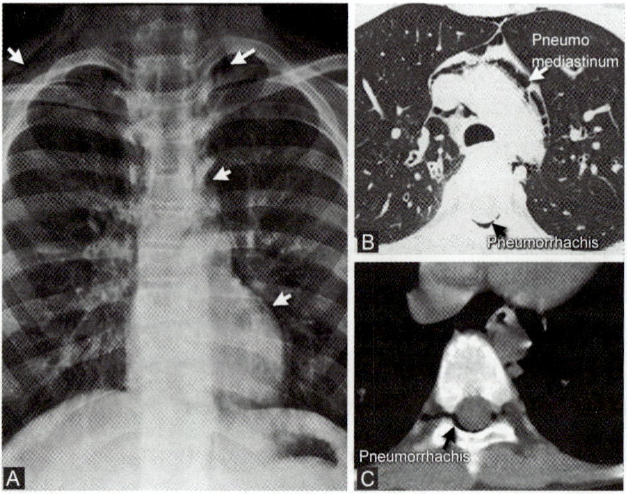

Figures 2.3A to C: This 14-year-old boy suffering from acute exacerbation of bronchial asthma. A—X-ray-Chest shows pneumomediastinum, pneumopericardium and subcutaneous emphysema (arrows). B and C—Axial CT chest shows pneumopericardium and pneumorrhachis.

POST TRAUMATIC PSEUDOMENINGOCELE

Avulsion injuries of the brachial plexus result in contusion or transaction of a nerve root, generally at its attachment to the spinal cord. These injuries are as a result of stretching of nerve root beyond its endurance in motorcycle and bicycle accidents. These injuries are because of distracting forces tearing the arachnoid and dural sheath of the nerve root and CSF extends along the course of the torn nerve root and along the epidural space with resultant pseudomeningocele. They often involve the lower cervical region (Figures 2.4A and B).

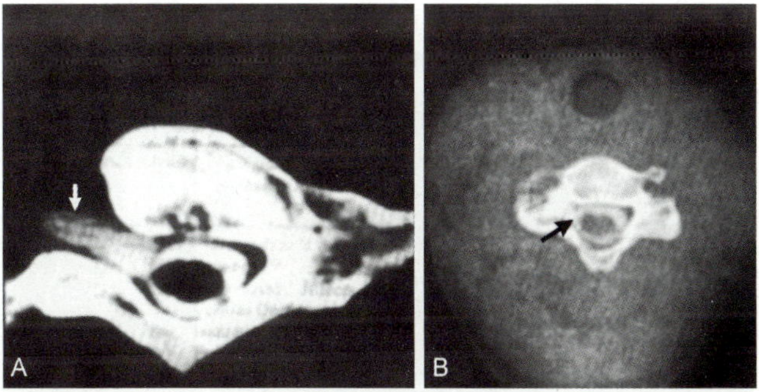

Figures 2.4A and B: A 15-year-old boy, following a fall from a bicycle two months ago presented with loss of movement of right upper limb associated with loss of sensation along lateral aspect of upper limb. CT myelography (CTM) of cervical spine revealed a bulbous out-pouching emerging from the right side neural foramen C5—6 (A) in both frontal and lateral projections and diagnosed as post traumatic pseudomeningocele extending over a length of 1.85 cm.

NEUROFIBROMA

Nerofibroma arises from non-specific cells in the nerve sheath. It is a benign expansile lesion through which the nerve passes. When it grows in size it enlarges the foramina through which it passes or contiguous bones undergo pressure erosion leading to bony defect. On MRI, neurofibromas have intermediate signal intensity on T1-weighted images, very high signal intensity on T2-weighted images and following gadolinium enhancement (Figures 2.5A to D).

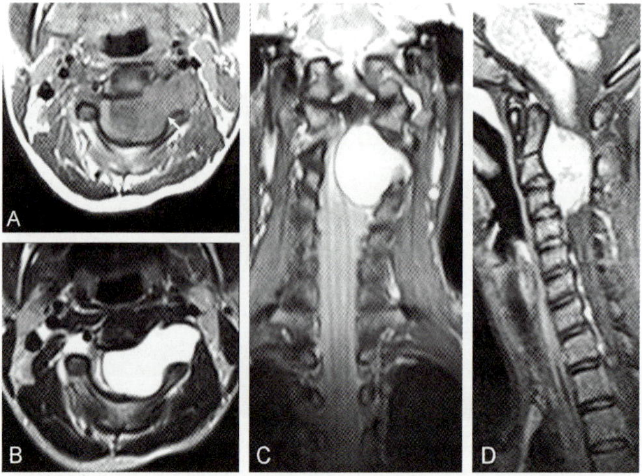

Figures 2.5A to D: A well defined dumb-bell shaped lesion is seen in the spinal canal, left neural foramen and left paraspinal region. The left neural foramen is widened. It is hypointense on T1 (A), hyperintense on T2 (B) and shows moderate homogeneous enhancement on postcontrast T1W images (D). Coronal T2W (C) image reveals compression and displacement of the cord to right.

NEUROBLASTOMA

Neuroblastoma is the most common extracranial pediatric neoplasm and the third most common pediatric malignancy after leukemia and CNS tumors. In the first year of life, neuroblastoma accounts for 50% of all tumors. Neuroblastomas can arise from anywhere along the sympathetic chain. Neuroblastomas arise from primitive neural crest cells that differentiate to form the sympathetic nervous system. Neuroblastomas consist predominantly of neuroblasts, whereas ganglioneuromas are composed entirely of well-differentiated cells (Figures 2.6A to H).

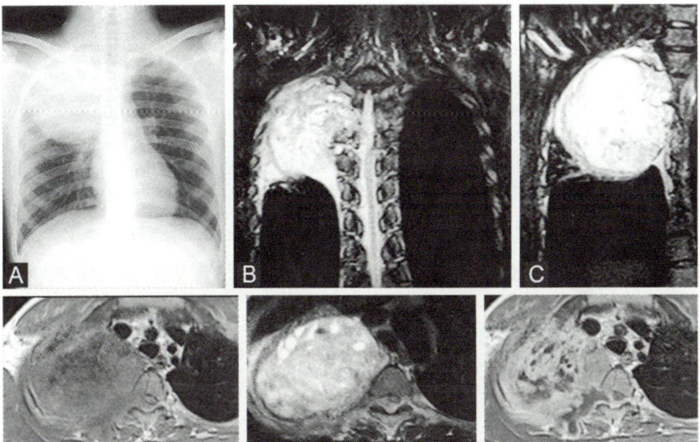

Figures 2.6A to F: Plain radiograph of chest (A) reveals a large well defined lesion in the right upper hemithorax. STIR Coronal images (B and C) reveal a heterogeneous hyperintense lesion in the paraspinal region with a small intra-spinal extension. It appears hypointense on T1W (D) image and shows heterogeneous enhancement on post-contrast axial T1W images (F).

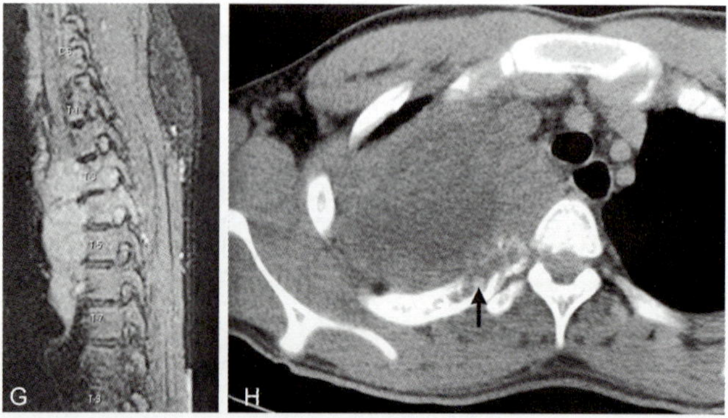

Figures 2.6G and H: Sagittal postcontrast T1W (G) image reveals enhancement of the vertebral bodies and their pedicles. Partial destruction of the adjacent rib is demonstrated on axial CT scan image (H).

SACROCOCCYGEAL TERATOMA

Sacrococcygeal teratoma is the most common solid neoplasm in neonates. It can be diagnosed prenatally by fetal ultrasound; however MRI is more accurate and reveals the intrapelvic and abdominal extent of the tumor. Treatment is complete surgical resection (Figures 2.7A to E).

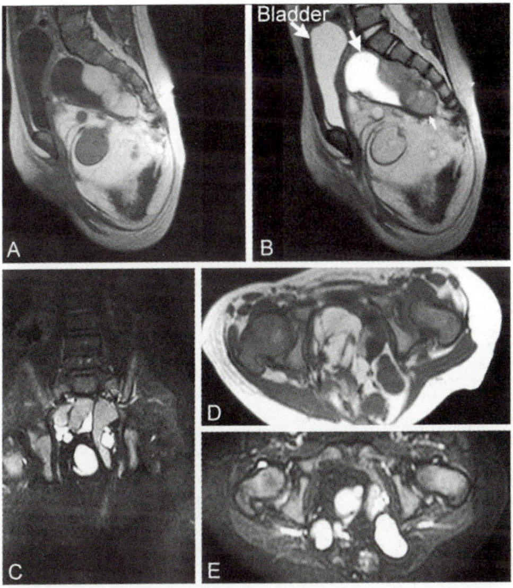

Figures 2.7A to E: Sagittal T1W (A), Sagittal T2W (B), Coronal STIR (C), Axial T1W (D) and Axial Fatsat (E) images of a one year old girl with buttock swelling since birth and difficulty during walking. Large well defined heterogeneous lesion is seen in the pelvis, posterior and inferior to the bladder. It is predominantly fatty with cystic and soft tissue components. The fatty component is suppressed on fatsat images (C and E) and the cystic component is hyperintense on T2W images. There is no intraspinal extension.

CHAPTER

Three

Paranasal Sinuses Face and Neck

Parvez Sheik
Amol Sasane

BRANCHIAL CLEFT CYST

Branchial cleft cyst is the most common cyst to arise in the neck and the most common congenital mass of the lateral neck. Othes masses include thyroglossal duct cyst, ectopic thymic cyst, lymphangioma, dermoid and epidermoid cyst. Cross-sectional imaging is the mainstay of diagnosis for these lesions (Figures 3.1A to D).

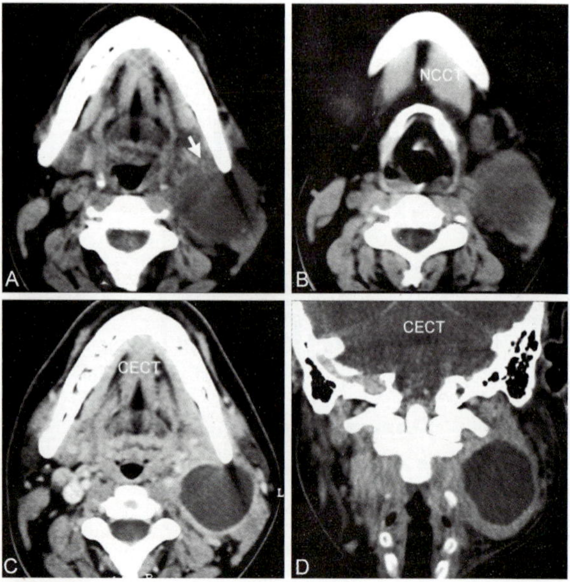

Figures 3.1A to D: Second branchial cleft cyst in a 16-year-old male with painless cystic swelling on left side of neck.

CYSTIC HYGROMA

Cystic hygroma is *benign, congenital* multiloculated *lymphatic* lesion that can arise anywhere, but is classically found in the left *posterior triangle* of the *neck*. It can be *disfiguring* (Figures 3.2A and B).

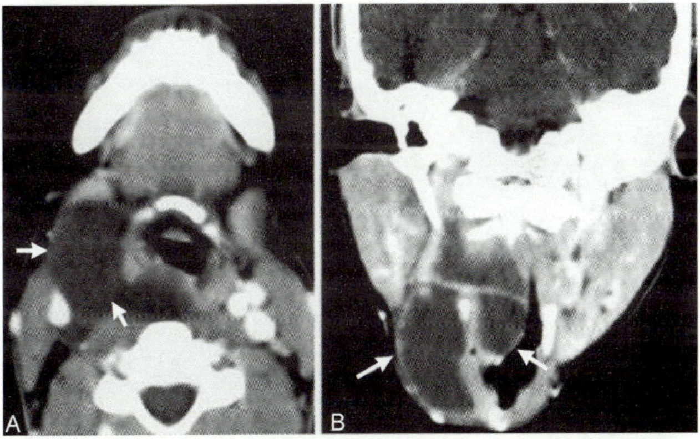

Figures 3.2A and B: A—Cystic hygroma mass is seen insinuating in the right retropharyngeal and parapharyngeal spaces, displacing the carotid space laterally. B—Cyst shows internal septae but no solid component.

CT GUIDED SCLEROTHERAPY IN CYSTIC HYGROMA

Cystic hygroma is a lymphangioma developing in the connective tissues. CT guided sclerotherapy with sodium tetradecyl sulphate is found to be effective (Figures 3.3A to D).

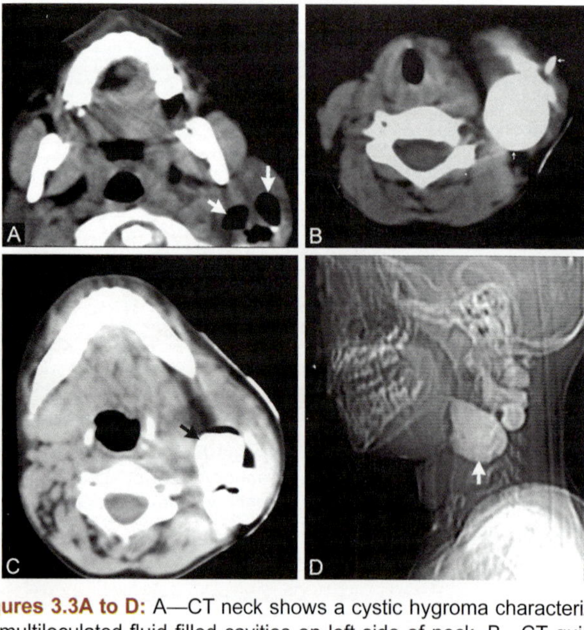

Figures 3.3A to D: A—CT neck shows a cystic hygroma characterized by multiloculated fluid filled cavities on left side of neck. B—CT guided sclerotherapy with sodium tetradecyl sulphate (shown by vertical arrow). Site of injection is shown by horizontal arrow. C—Sclerosant is seen filling almost entire lesion. D—Post sclerotherapy film showing extent of the spread of sclerosant.

INTERNAL JUGULAR PHLEBECTASIA

Varicose veins are a common venous anomaly, whereas phlebectasia is rare. It is an abnormal dilation of an isolated vein. Any vein may be affected and the condition is usually asymptomatic. Internal jugular phlebectasia is abnormal dilation of internal jugular vein.

It presents as a soft fluctuant and fusiform swelling lying in the anterior aspect of the lower part of the neck which changes in size and becomes visible and prominent during coughing, crying, sneezing, straining or during the Valsalva maneuvers. The swelling closely mimics the signs of either a laryngocele or a pharyngocele (Figures 3.4A and B).

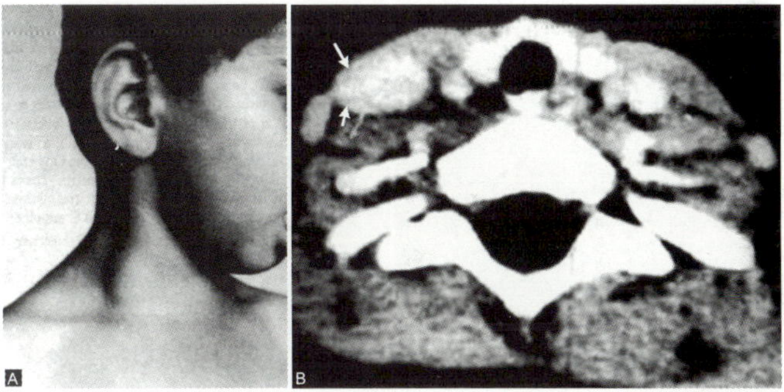

Figures 3.4A and B: A—Swelling in the neck seen only while coughing. B—CT Scan at the level of thyroid shows gross dilatation of the right internal jugular vein (arrow) as compared to that on the left. Diagnosis is internal jugular phlebectasia.

PAROTID ABSCESS

The look of parotid abscess varies depending on the amount of liquefaction that has occurred. In the early stages the gland is enlarged; hypoechoic area within the parenchyma of the gland may be seen; later a thick wall is formed at the periphery with anechoic central area, septations and internal echoes may be seen. On Doppler, no color flow is seen centrally in the abscess, the periphery may show vascularity indicating its inflammatory nature (Figures 3.5A to B). Intraluminal hyperechoic calculi in the Stensen's duct may be seen on ultrasound.

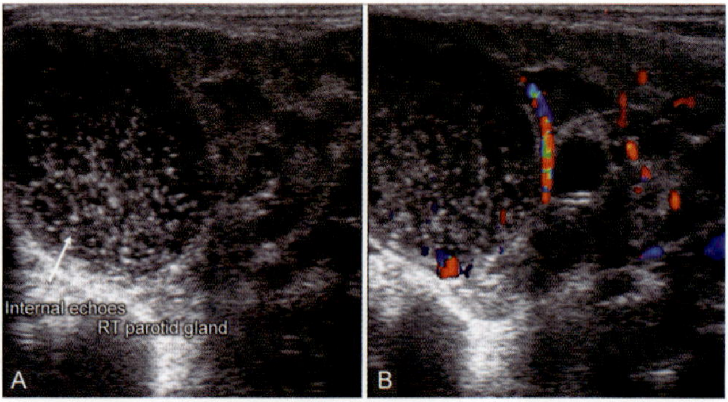

Figures 3.5A and B: Parotid USG shows a large, well-defined hypoechoic area within the parenchyma of the gland with internal echoes. On Doppler, no color flow is seen centrally, the periphery shows vascularity indicating its inflammatory nature.

FOREIGN BODY EAR

Foreign objects in the ear are common, especially in children. Most foreign bodies get stuck in the external auditory canal and are often placed by the patients themselves; the most common foreign objects are beads, beans, paper, cotton swabs, pebbles, insects etc. Insects can fly or crawl into the canal, leading to a frightening event as the insect's buzzing and movement is very loud and at times, irritant and painful (Figures 3.6A to B).

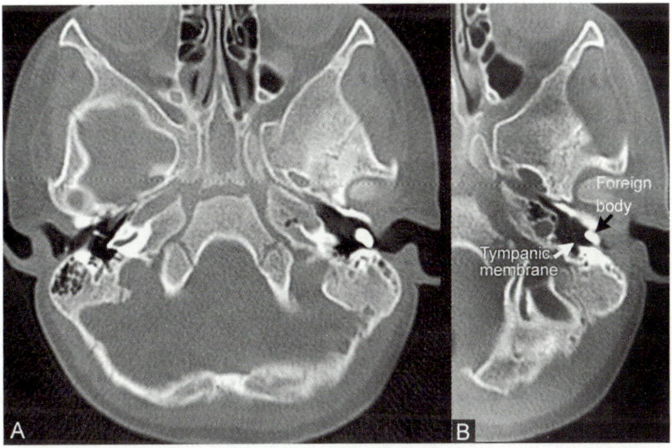

Figures 3.6A to B: Three-year-old girl while playing accidentally lodges a small pebble into the ear which is lying in external auditory canal as a foreign body.

ECTOPIC THYROID

Ectopic thyroid tissue can be found anywhere in the neck or tongue and the normal cervical position of the thyroid gland. It occurs most commonly at the base of tongue, identified as lingual, followed by sublingual and the anterior midline of neck. It is recommended to performing a thyroid scan in every case of thyroid ectopia to accurately identify all sites of functioning thyroid tissue (Figures 3.7A to F).

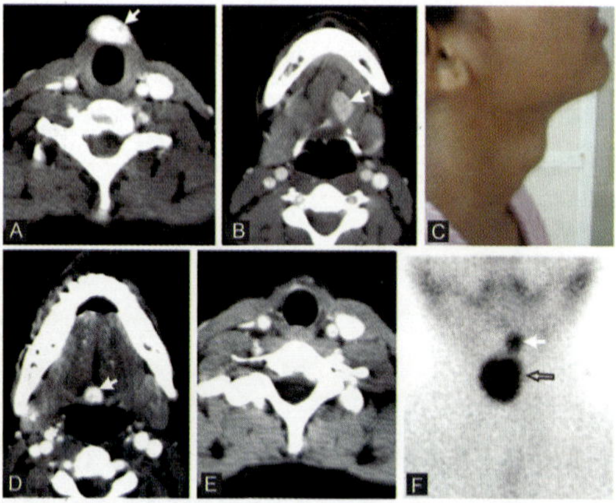

Figures 3.7A to F: Contrast CT in a 15-year-old girl with no complaints except for an anterior midline neck swelling (C), shows a triple ectopic thyroid as hyperdense intense enhancing soft masses at three places: at the posterior most part of tongue measuring 10x11x10 mm (D), at base of tongue on left side measuring 17x10x12 mm (B) and in the anterior midline of neck just below the hyoid bone measuring 15x24x26 mm (A). No thyroid gland is seen at normal position (E). F—Thyroid nuclear scan with 3 mCi technetium shows that no thyroid tissue is visualized in the normal location. Tracer uptake is seen in clinically palpable nodule (block arrow) and another small focus (arrow) of tracer uptake is seen above clinically palpable nodule, i.e. at the base of tongue.

RETINOBLASTOMA

Retinoblastoma arises from primitive neuroectodermal cells in retina. It may be hereditary or sporadic and may be bilateral. Over 80% of retinoblastoma shows evidence of calcification on CT scan. In patients under three years of age in whom a retinoblastoma is suspected, the presence of calcification on CT scan is virtually diagnostic (Figure 3.8).

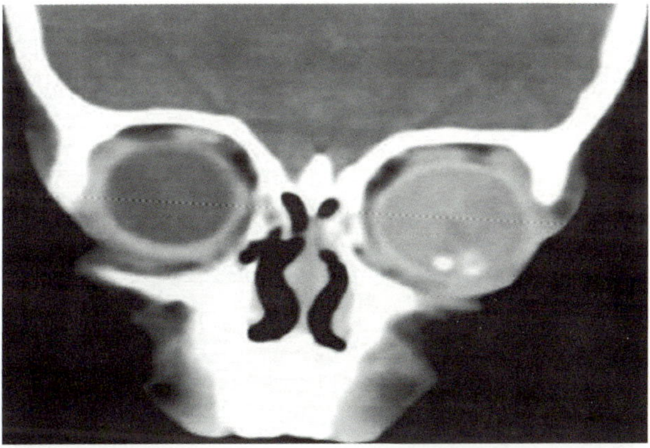

Figure 3.8: Two-year-old boy with proptosis left eye. Contrast CT orbits revealed calcification in the enhancing retinal soft tissue mass.

CHAPTER

Four

Chest and Mediastinum

Hariqbal Singh

KARTAGENER'S SYNDROME

Kartagener syndrome is *situs inversus* (reversal of the internal organs) accompanied by *bronchiectasis and chronic sinusitis.* Most cases are observed before the age of 15 years. Aetiology is unknown with autosomal recessive inheritance. Symptoms and sign are dyspnea, productive cough, recurrent respiratory infection and cold, pneumonia, rheumatoid arthritis, anosmia and clubbing of fingers (Figures 4.1A to F).

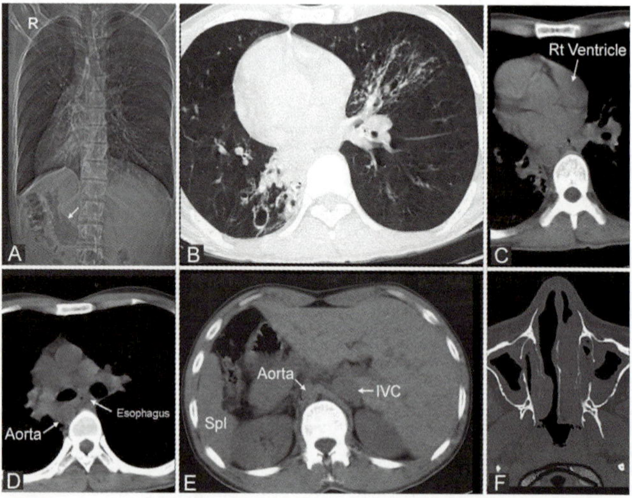

Figures 4.1A to F: A—X-ray shows situs inversus with heart and stomach (arrow) on the right side; B to D—Axial CT chest shows bronchiectasis, dextrocardia wirh morphologic right ventricle on the left and the left ventricle on the right; E—Plain axial CT at the level of renals shows liver and IVC on the left and the spleen and aorta on the right; F—Axial CT PNS shows chronic sinusitis in an individual with Kartagener syndrome.

EVENTRATION

Eventration of Diaphragm

In eventration of the diaphragm it is permanently elevated and retains its continuity and attachments to the costal margins. It is seldom symptomatic and often requires no treatment. It often presents in the neonatal period with respiratory distress. However, this condition may be confused with a traumatic rupture of the diaphragm in a patient with trauma (Figures 4.2A and B).

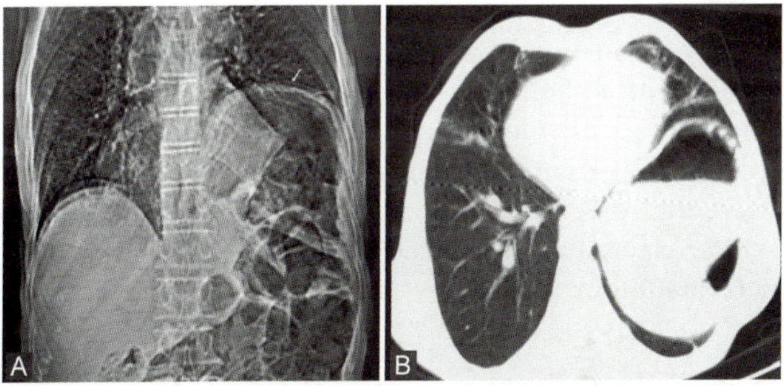

Figures 4.2A and B: A—Scanogram shows elevated left hemidiaphragm; B—Axial CT chest shows stomach with oral contrast extending into chest.

BRONCHOCELE

Contrast enhanced CT scan showing non-enhancing fluid attenuating lesion seen in the right upper lobe appears to be within the dilated bronchi of posterior segment of right upper lobe. Can be better appreciated on coronal reformatted image (Figures 4.3A and B).

Bronchocele is commonly seen in congenital bronchial atresia, where there is fluid accumulation in the bronchus, distal to the atretic segment of bronchus. There are other causes for bronchocele like carcinoids obstructing the segmental bronchus.

X-ray chest is the first investigation to be done and suspected on it. Spiral CT is the examination of choice, not only to show all the components of the anomaly and to estimate the extent of air trapping but also for ruling out differential diagnosis such as bronchogenic cyst, bronchiectasis, aspergillosis, completely thrombosed arteriovenous malformation or pulmonary aneurysms and tumors.

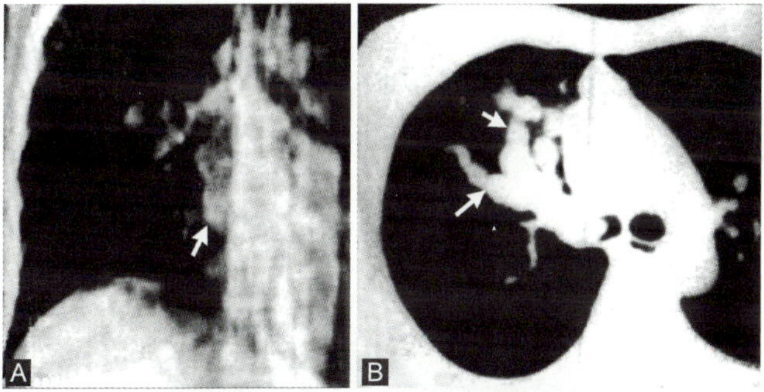

Figures 4.3A and B: A—Chest topogram shows bronchocele seen as rounded parahilar opacity; B—CT scan chest shows bronchocele as sacccular dilatation radiating from the right hilum. A soft tissue mass is seen protruding into the right main bronchus.

THORACIC NEUROBLASTOMA

Some neuroblastomas are known to undergo spontaneous regression (Figures 4.4A and B) or induced differentiation to benign ganglioneuroma.

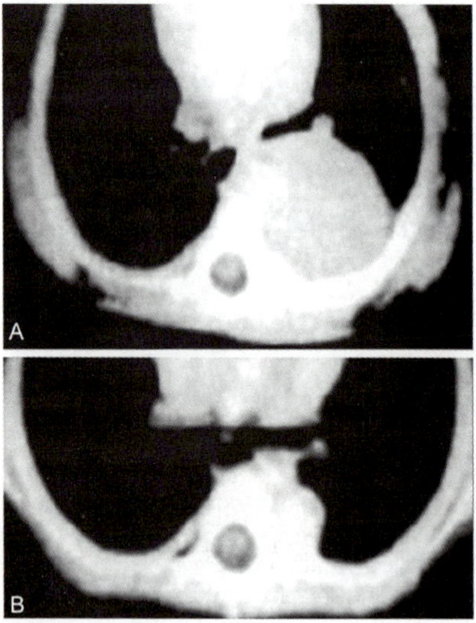

Figures 4.4A and B: (A) Posterior mediastinal mass seen incidentally on chest roentgenogram in a 6-week-old female infant. CT chest at the level of main bronchi demonstrates posterior mediastinal mass 3x3 cm histologically confirmed as neuroblastoma seen lifting the left main bronchus and the left pulmonary artery which is seen as a nipple like small nodule without infiltrations into the surrounding tissue. (B) CT scan 3 months later, section at the same level shows marked spontaneous regression of lesion to 8 mm size.

TUBERCULOUS EFFUSIONS

Diseases of the pericardium are clearly visualized on CT. It detects pericardial effusion thickening of the pericardium and calcification with a high degree of sensitivity and specificity and is an accurate method of demonstrating the extent and distribution of pericardial calcification. CT also demonstrates the presence of additional finding of pleural effusion or ascites (Figures 4.5A and B).

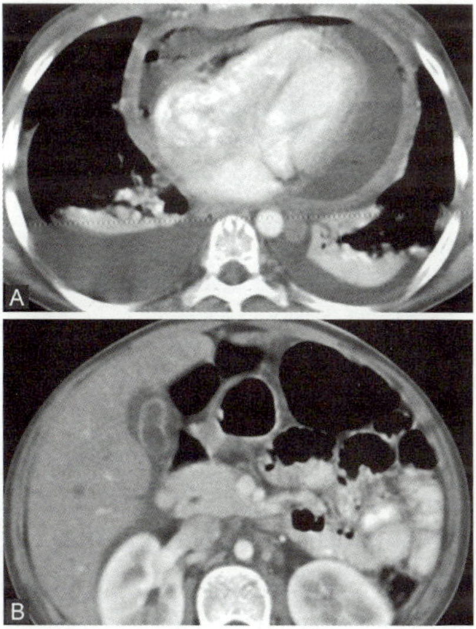

Figures 4.5A and B: Pericardial effusion, pleural effusion and ascites in a 13-year-old female. A—CT chest shows pericardial effusion with few air pockets (post drainage), the fluid thickness is up to 25 mm, outer layer of pericardium is thickened. Bilateral pleural effusion is present; B—Free fluid is present in the perihepatic and paracolic gutters and pericholecystic area.

COARCTATION OF AORTA

In coarctation of aorta there is a characteristic shelf-like narrowing of the aorta which usually occurs just beyond the origin of the left subclavian artery. The severity of coarctation or narrowing can vary considerably and it is this severity which determines the age of presentation (Figures 4.6A to D and 4.7A to C).

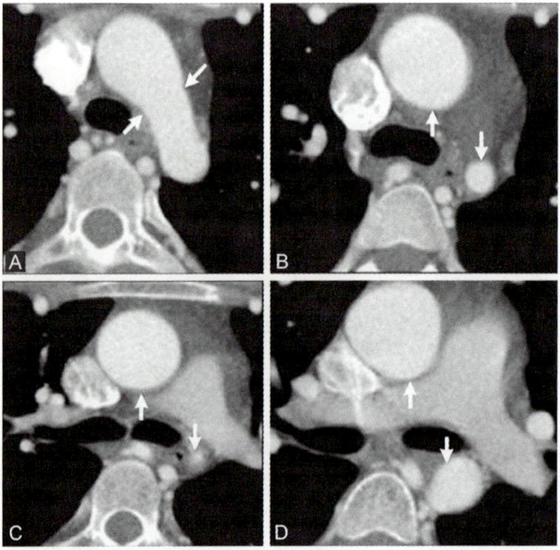

Figures 4.6A to D: CT Aortic Angiography in a case of post-ductal coarctation of aorta. (A) Aortic arch shows reduction in diameter of descending aorta as compared to ascending. (B and C) The diameter of ascending aorta (upright arrow) is maintained but that of descending aorta (down pointing arrow) has abruptly reduced. (D) Descending aorta returns to normal caliber.

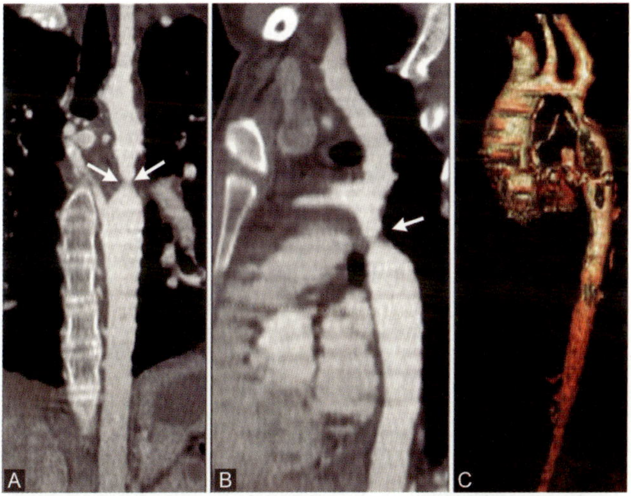

Figures 4.7A to C: A and B—Coronal and sagittal reformatted image shows the actual site of coarctation. C—Color coded CT angiogram shows exact location of narrowing.

CHAPTER
Five

Abdomen

Hariqbal Singh
Anand Kamat
Sheetal Dhote

GASTROINTESTINAL TRACT

Eventration with Malrotation of Midgut

Elevation of a single hemidiaphragm is usually secondary to adjacent pleural, pulmonary, subphrenic disease or due to phrenic nerve palsy. Rarely it is related to an intrinsic weakness of the diaphragm. In eventration weakened diaphragmatic muscles results in the upward displacement of abdominal contents but its incidence with malrotation of midgut is not seen. Occasionally it is associated with superior renal ectopia as the kidney continues to migrate beyond the normal renal fossa during development and ends up in the thorax.

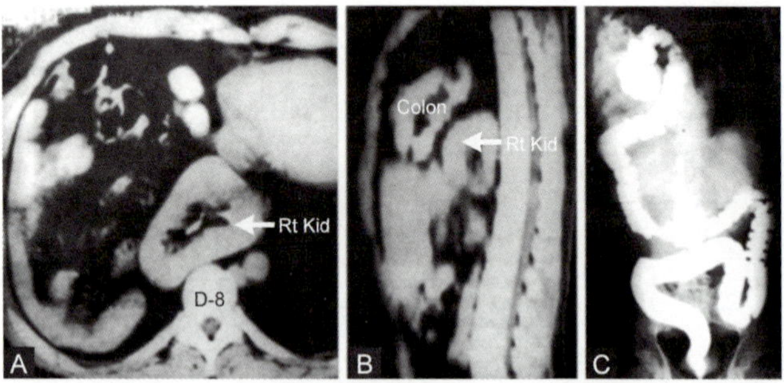

Figures 5.1A to C: A—Axial CECT at chest level, B—Sagittal reconstruction of chest and abdomen shows eventration of right hemidiaphragm with right kidney migrating into chest at D8 vertebral level. C—Barium enema examination shows redundancy of the colon with ascending colon and cecum extending into the right hemithorax underlying the right hemidiaphragm. Upper GIT study (not in the figure) demonstrated the stomach in normal position with duodenojejunal flexure on the right side as part of malrotation of right gut.

Duodenal Esophageal Atresia

Esophageal and duodenal atresia have characteristic appearances on ultrasound, babies with duodenal atresia have slight distension of the upper abdomen as the stomach can decompress through the esophagus. When esophageal atresia coexists with duodenal atresia, the stomach and duodenum are dilated due to the trapped gastric secretions. The abnormal degree of dilation allows discrimination from duodenal atresia.

Newborn baby presented with distended and palpable masses in upper abdomen with inability to pass a nasogastric tube. The kidigram shows gasless abdomen with coiling of nasogastric tube in upper thoracic region suggesting esophageal atresia. Ultrasound of abdomen shows fluid-filled stomach and duodenum. The ultrasound appearances suggest duodenal atresia associated with esophageal atresia. Laparotomy confirmed the findings and duodeno-duodenostomy was carried out followed by esophageal repair at a later date (Figures 5.2A to G).

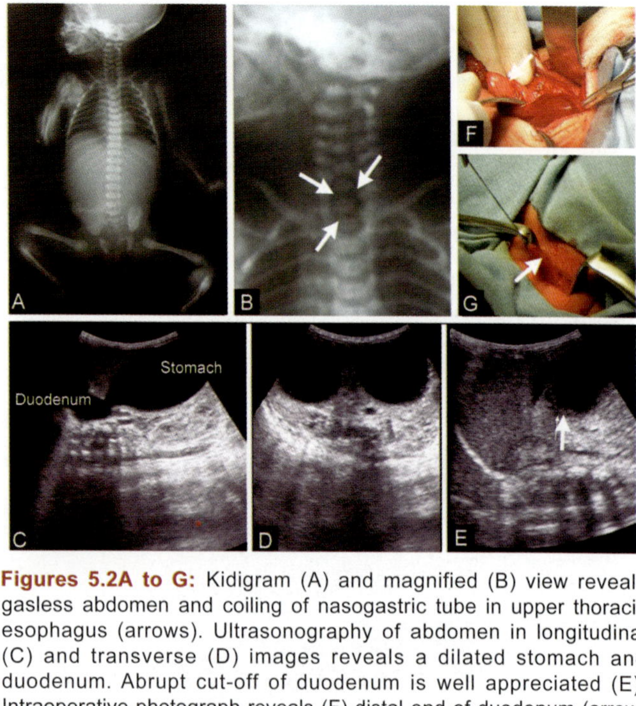

Figures 5.2A to G: Kidigram (A) and magnified (B) view reveals gasless abdomen and coiling of nasogastric tube in upper thoracic esophagus (arrows). Ultrasonography of abdomen in longitudinal (C) and transverse (D) images reveals a dilated stomach and duodenum. Abrupt cut-off of duodenum is well appreciated (E). Intraoperative photograph reveals (F) distal end of duodenum (arrow) and (G) blind end of esophagus (arrow).

Epigastric Hernia

Typical locations of epigastric hernia are the points of weakness where no muscle is present, along the linea alba in the midline. On ultrasound, seen in cross section, herniated bowel loops appear as target lesions with strong reflective central echoes representing air in the lumen; when obstructed, they appear as tubular fluid-filled structures containing valvulae conniventes or fecal material. Omentum may also herniate through the defect in anterior abdominal wall (Figure 5.3). Congenital epigastric hernias are gastrochisis and omphalocele.

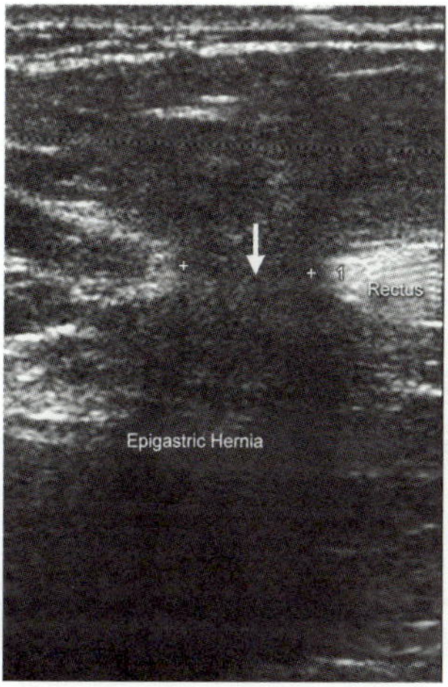

Figure 5.3: Ultrasound shows a rent in anterior abdominal wall (arrow), forming a neck which is displacing the *rectus abdominis* muscle. The herniated sac with contents is appreciated.

Gastroschisis

Gastroschisis is congenital epigastric hernias. It is a full thickness defect of the anterior abdominal wall, usually located to the right of umbilical cord. The defect is generally small and herniated organs include bowel loops and rarely liver. The other congenital epigastric hernias omphalocele (Figure 5.4).

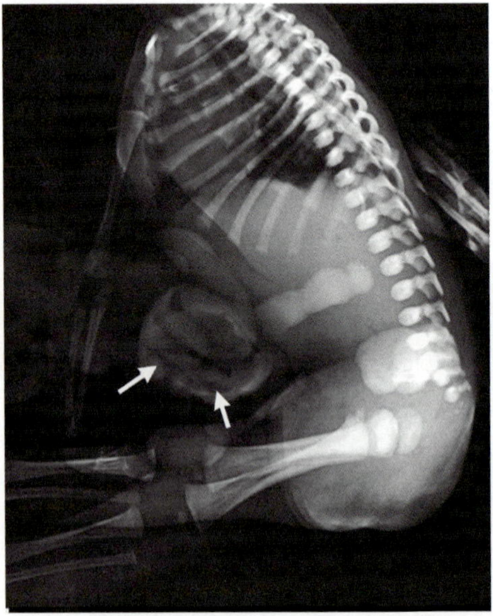

Figure 5.4: Kidigram shows gastroschisis with herniation of bowel loops.

Hirschsprung's Disease

Hirschsprung's disease is due to arrest in the normal cranial-to-caudal neural cell migration, resulting in absence of ganglion cells within the myenteric plexus of the bowel wall. 70% of cases involve the rectosigmoid region. There is male predominance (4:1) in rectosigmoid region. A discrete zone of transition with a change in caliber of the bowel is more often seen in children than in the neonatal period (Figures 5.5A and B).

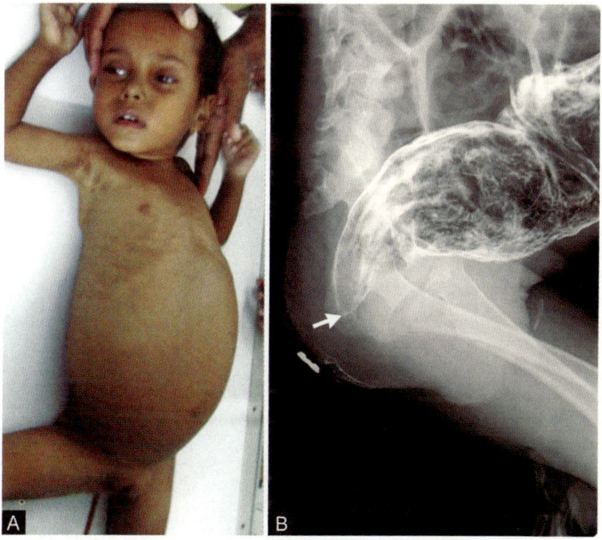

Figures 5.5A and B: Barium enema examination shows a discrete zone of transition (arrow) with abrupt increase in caliber of bowel in 5-year-old male presented with gross abdominal distension and failure to pass stool since a week.

LIVER

Hepatic Hemangioma

The need for USG contrast arises when the lesions are isoechoic to the background parenchyma or are diffusely isoechoic and are difficult to pick up or be characterized by B mode ultrasound. Therefore, the use of USG contrast has significantly changed the capability of ultrasound imaging. 17-year-old male reported with general weakness, was subjected to ultrasound followed by contrast enhanced scan with SONOVUE by BRACCO (Figures 5.6A to E).

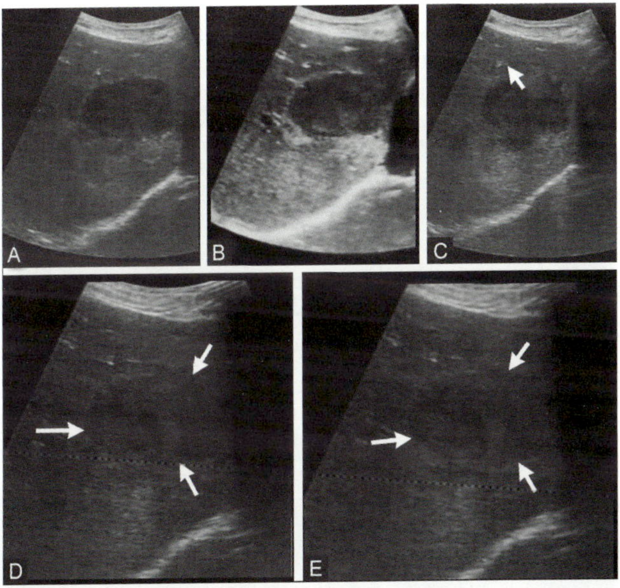

Figures 5.6A to E: A—On ultrasound right lobe of liver shows a well defined hyoechoic lesion; B—Intravenous contrast injected, in arterial phase shows outlining the edges of the lesion seen as increased echogenicity of the margins of the lesion; C—Gradually the circulating contrast shows early filling-up the lesion more in the anterior aspect. As a result of peripheral filling, there is some change in shape and outline of the lesion; D and E—Show excellent filling of the lesion resulting in echogenicity isodense to the hepatic tissue which was hyoechoic in precontrast image (A).

Hepatoblastoma

Hepatoblastoma is the most common primary liver tumor in children, accounting for 79% of pediatric liver malignancies in children younger than 15 years (Figure 5.7).

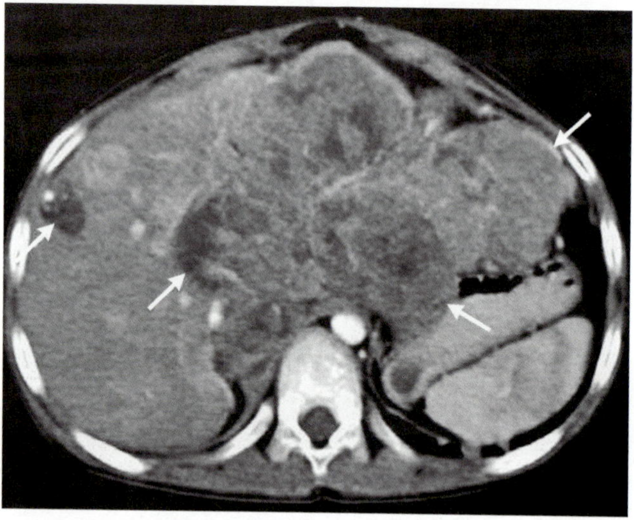

Figure 5.7: 12-year-old male with pain in abdomen and fever since 20 days diagnosed on CT as hepatoblastoma.

Gallbladder in Hepatitis

In hepatitis, gallbladder frequently shows non-specific changes like thickening of gallbladder wall > 3 mm, multiple focal noncontiguous hypoechoic pockets of edema, fluid within the thickened wall can be seen (Figures 5.8A and B). Other changes can be a thin rim of fluid representing edema in the wall, a double wall appearance or presence of sludge in the gallbladder cavity.

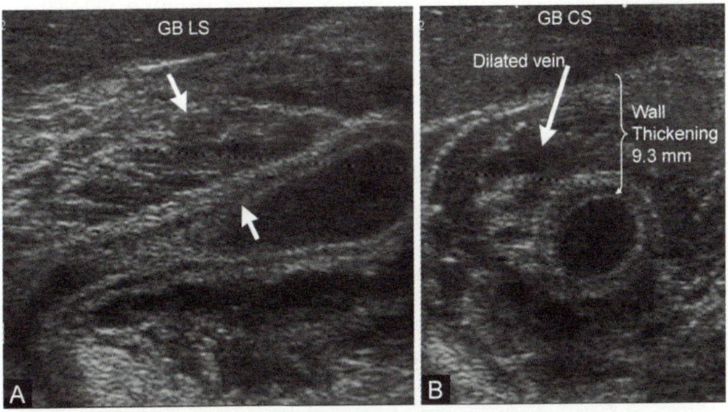

Figures 5.8A and B: Gallbladder shows gross thickening of the wall (between the arrows in (A) due to edema and dilated veins seen within the wall (B) in a four-year-old child with hepatitis.

Choledochal Cyst

The origin of these cysts is uncertain. The most likely etiology is bile duct injury resulting from sequelae of an anomalous junction of the pancreatic duct and the distal common bile duct (CBD). This anomalous junction results in chronic reflux of pancreatic enzymes into the biliary tree with resultant weakening, scarring and dilatation of the CBD wall. Complications associated with choledochal cyst include cholelithiasis, choledocholithiasis, cystolithiasis, ascending cholangitis, bile duct strictures, intrahepatic abscesses, biliary cirrhosis, portal hypertension and hepatobiliary malignancy. The large choledochal cysts can be confused with large intrahepatic cystic lesions such as hydatid cyst on axial CT imaging alone (Figures 5.9A to E).

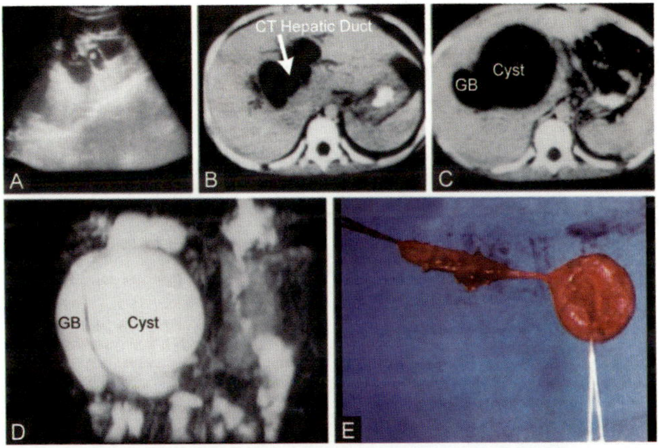

Figures 5.9A to E: A—US shows the dilated, tortuous and ectatic left hepatic duct; B—CECT demonstrates a large cyst lying medial to gallbladder; C—CECT shows the dilated, tortuous and ectatic left hepatic duct (similar to USG Figure A) with minimal dilatation of intrahepatic biliary radicles; D—MRI cholangiography shows the cyst medial to the gallbladder with dilated left hepatic duct; E—Photograph of resected specimen shows choledochal cyst, gallbladder and the cystic duct.

SPLEEN

Splenunculus

Splenunculus or accessory spleen is congenital nodule, composed of normal splenic tissue. The *spleen* forms from multiple smaller components during embryogenesis, and failure of this fusion leads to one or more nodules or splenunculi remaining separate. They are *extraperitoneal,* benign and asymptomatic and should not be confused with *splenosis* which is acquired and intraperitoneal (Figures 5.10A and B).

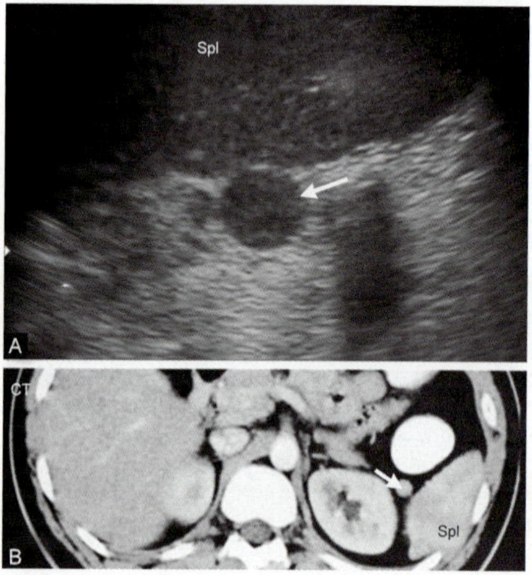

Figures 5.10A and B: A—Ultrasound image shows a small round structure medial to spleen (arrow), the splenunculus. It has same echo signatures as spleen; B—Contrast CT images show a small round structure medial to spleen, the splenunculus. It has same density as spleen.

KIDNEY

Duplication of Ureter

The duplication of ureter may be incomplete (the ureters fusing at some point in their course and having a common distal orifice) or complete (both ureters having separate distal orifices). Incomplete duplication is almost always of no clinical significance. Although in a small proportion of cases it may be associated with yo-yo reflux in which urine from one ureter refluxes back up the other ureter. This may lead to loin pain on micturition and urinary tract infection (Figures 5.11A to G).

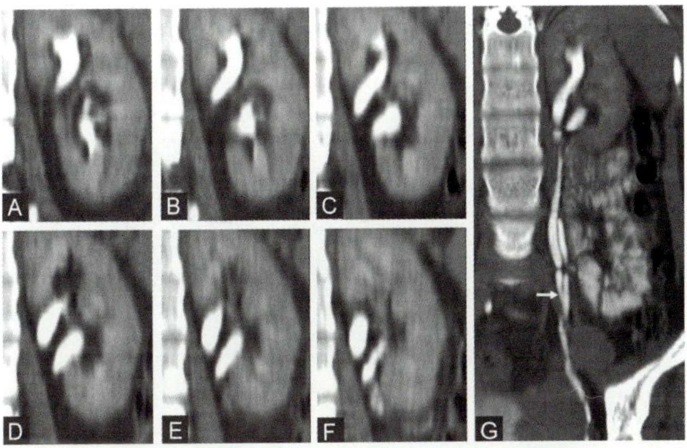

Figures 5.11A to G: Intravenous urogram shows left kidney (A to C), two pelvicalyceal collecting systems, twin pelvis and ureter seen in D to F. G is coronal reconstruction, shows left kidney with twin collecting system and two ureters which unite at L4 level.

Left Renal Aplasia

Renal aplasia is the predominant cause of congenital solitary kidneys. Congenital solitary kidney, which is susceptible to renal failure, has been considered mostly due to unilateral renal agenesis and partly due to renal aplasia. Risk of familial recurrence and of other associated anomalies is known to be much higher in renal agenesis than in renal aplasia. However, differential diagnosis between the two renal anomalies is difficult, and renal agenesis has been found much less frequently in ultrasound screening studies of fetuses than in autopsy studies (Figures 5.12A and B).

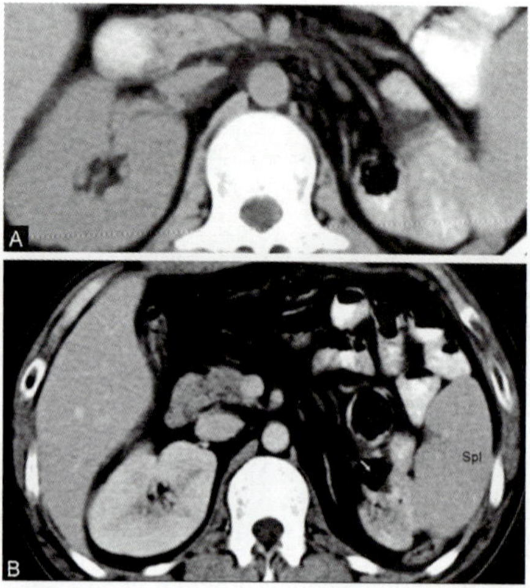

Figures 5.12A and B: A (plain) and B (contrast)—CT images show absence of left kidney. The left renal fossa is occupied by intestinal loops.

Retrocaval Ureter

Retrocaval ureter is a congenital anomaly. Common presentations are right lumbar pain, dull aching or intermittent (renal colic), recurrent urinary tract infections and microscopic or gross hematuria. There is a high incidence of calculi due to stasis. Diagnosis is confirmed by ultrasonography and intravenous urography. Spiral CT scan and MRI help sometimes to delineate the anatomy clearly and non-invasively (Figures 5.13A and B).

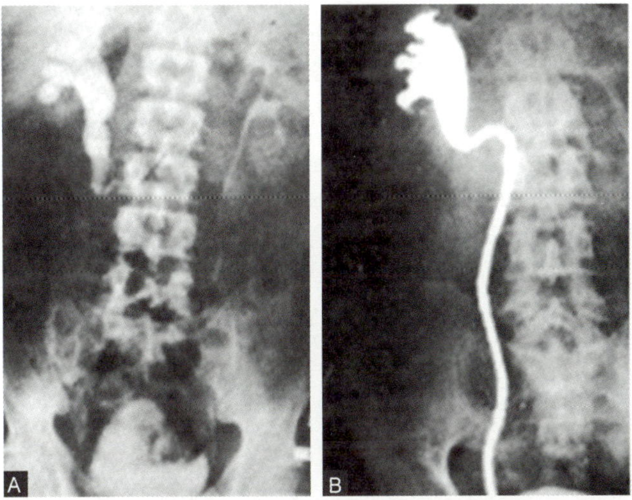

Figures 5.13A and B: A—IVP shows dilated right upper ureter, and upper third ureter shows S shaped curvature towards the midline. B—RGP shows upper third of right ureter curving towards the midline (arrow).

Posterior Urethral Valves with Cystitis

Cystitis in children, frequently results in upper urinary tract infection (UTI) which is most often due to bacterial infection. Difference between lower UTI (cystitis) and upper UTI (pyelonephritis) is difficult in small children and rarely crucial. Imaging algorithm will be similar in both situations, an important aspect being to exclude outflow obstruction and presence of vesicoureteric reflux.

Posterior urethral valves are the frequent cause of urethral obstruction in male children. These valves are positioned at the proximal urethra, the distal most portion of prostatic urethra resulting in obstruction in the flow of urine. The consequence is dilatation of prostatic urethra. The diagnostic study is micturating cystourethrogram (MCU), which should be carried out once infection is treated. MCU demonstrates dilated prostatic urethra and is treated by cystoscopic valve fulguration (Figure 5.14).

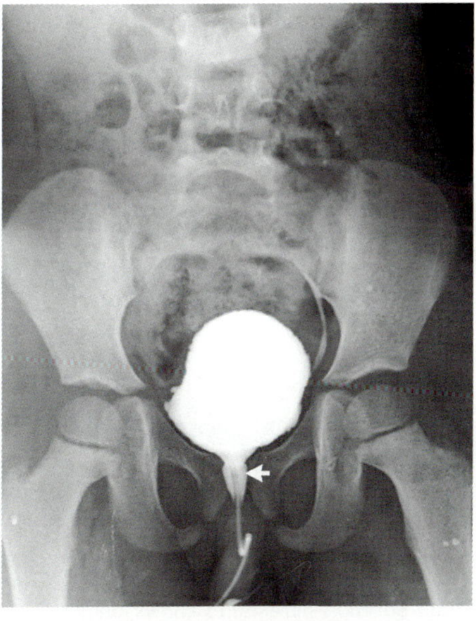

Figure 5.14: Micturating cystourethrogram shows dilatation of prostatic urethra secondary to posterior urethral valves with cystitis seen as irregularity of bladder wall.

Multicystic Dysplastic Kidney Disease

Ultrasonography allows demonstration of fetal kidneys and urinary bladder from second trimester and enables to detect major congenital anomalies of the urinary system. Multicystic dysplastic kidney disease (MCDKD) is usually an incidental finding during routine antenatal sonographic examination (Figures 5.15A to C). The incidence of MCDKD is about 1 in 10,000 births.

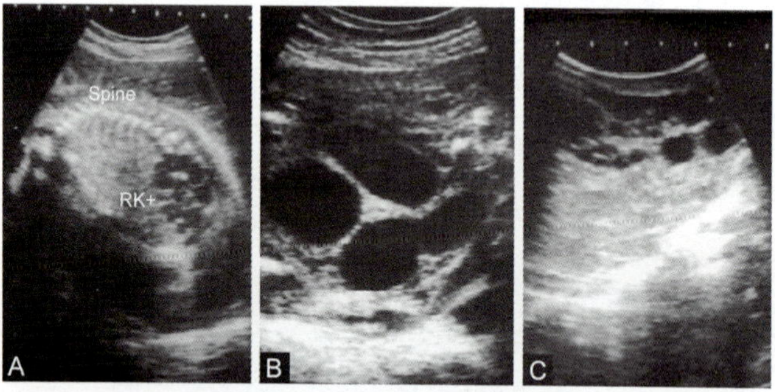

Figures 5.15A to C: A—Antenatal ultrasound shows enlarged right fetal kidney with multiple cysts; B—Ultrasound shows dilated bowel loops; C—Post abortion ultrasound shows enlarged kidneys with multiple cysts.

Polycystic Kidneys Disease (PKD)

PKD is an *autosomal dominant* trait and is much more common in adults. An *autosomal recessive* form of PKD also exists and appears in infancy or childhood. In early stages of the disease, the cysts cause the kidney to swell up (Figures 5.16A and B), disrupting kidney function and leading to chronic high blood pressure and kidney infections. Bleeding in a cyst can cause *flank pain*. *Kidney stones* are more common in PKD. PKD may be associated with brain *aneurysms*, cysts in the liver, pancreas, and *testes* and colonic d*iverticula*.

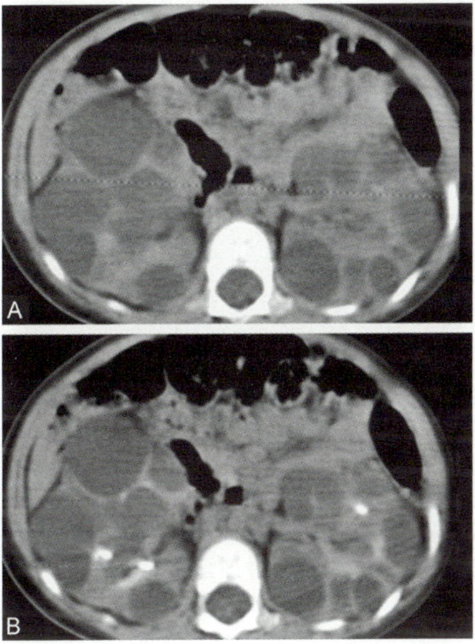

Figures 5.16A and B: Plain and contrast CT abdomen shows bilateral polycystic kidneys with parenchymal thinning and delayed excretion of contrast.

Obstructive Uropathy

Obstructive uropathy results in hydronephrosis and hydroureter depending on the site of mechanical obstruction. Hyronephrosis is dilation of the calyces and renal pelvis appearing on ultrasound as anechoic areas and gradually there is reduction in renal cortical thickness (Figures 5.17A and B). Ultrasound is a quick, safe and sensitive tool for detecting hydronephrosis and possibly the cause.

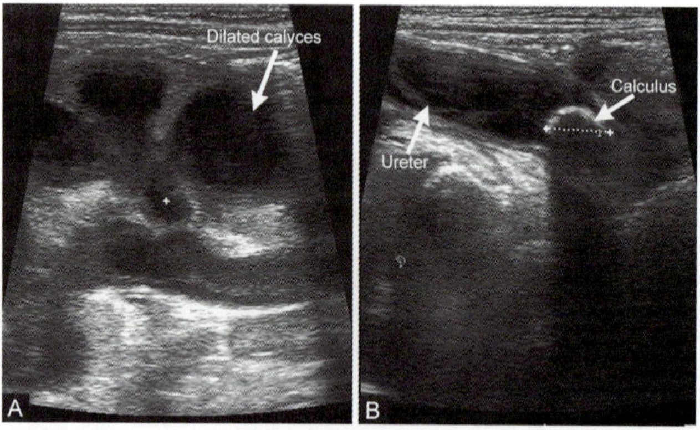

Figures 5.17A and B: A 9 mm diameter calculus is seen in proximal ureter (B) with acoustic shadowing and resultant hydronephrosis and hydroureter (A and B) with marked thinning of renal cortex. There is thickening of wall of ureter with internal echos in dilated ureter are suggestive of inflammatory process.

Wilms' Tumor (Nephroblastoma) with Hepatic and Pulmonary Metastasis

Wilms' tumor primarily affects children. Also known as nephroblastoma, it is the most common malignant tumor of the kidneys in children. The peak incidence of Wilms' tumor is 3 to 4 years of age and is rare after 6 years of age. Most Wilms' tumors can be cured (Figures 5.18A to D).

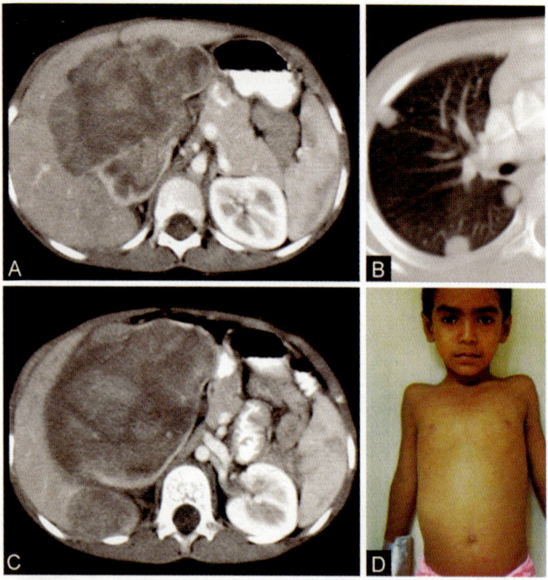

Figures 5.18A to D: A—CECT shows large well defined enhancing mass lesion 9×10 cm with few areas of necrosis, involving the right kidney, sparing its upper pole. Medially the lesion is seen to displace the pancreas and great vessels to left side with compression of IVC. Cranially the lesion is seen to abut the inferior surface of liver and inferiorly extent to iliac crest; C—Another 3x2.4 cm heterogeneously enhancing lesion is noted in posteroinferior segment of right lobe of liver is metastasis. Filling defect is noted in right renal vein which is stretched out and compression of IVC possibly tumor thrombosis; B—Multiple well defined metastatic lesions are seen in the lungs, seen in a six-year-old male child with gradually increasing lump abdomen (D).

Mullerian Duct Cyst

Mullerian duct cyst is an uncommon congenital anomaly. It is usually small, asymptomatic, midline, cystic lesion, located behind the superior half of the prostatic urethra and connected to the verumontanum by a thin stalk. Rarely a mullerian duct cyst may be associated with renal agenesis and hypospadias. MRI accurately defines anatomic relationship when one is planning to excise a mullerian duct cyst due to multiplanar imaging capacity, superior soft tissue contrast, and absence of ionizing radiation (Figures 5.19A to F).

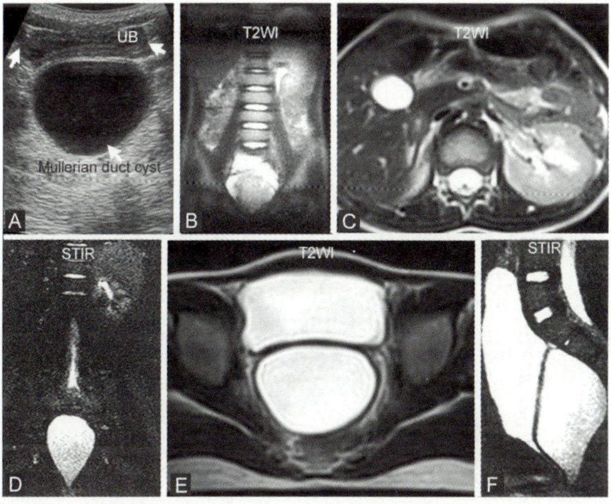

Figures 5.19A to F: In a five-year-old male child, transabdominal USG (A) shows cystic nature lesion posterior to bladder (arrows). Agenesis of right kidney with normal left kidney is seen in and coronal and axial T2 weighted images (B and C). Pear shaped cystic nature mass lesion seen hyperintense on STIR and T2 weighted images (D and E). Sagittal STIR MR image (F) shows that there is no communication between cystic lesion and urinary bladder.

Bladder Diverticula

CT scan of 14-year-old male with history of exstrophy of bladder (ectopia vesicae). Exstrophy of bladder is a congenital abnormality in which there is incomplete development or absence of the infra-umbilical part of the anterior abdominal wall, associated with incomplete development of the bladder. These cases often develop bladder diverticulae which are localized out-pouchings of the bladder mucosa between fibres of the detrusor muscles (pseudo-diverticulae) resulting from a congential or acquired defect in the bladder wall. A wide neck diverticulum fills and empties readily with the bladder, but in a narrow neck diverticulum there is poor emptying, the diverticulum may be better appreciated on post-void film.

Renal calculus disease is relatively uncommon in children. The etiology of renal calculi in children could be due to infection, developmental anomalies of the genitourinary tract or metabolic disorders. Non-contrast CT shows virtually all stones as high attenuation foci (Figures 5.20A to D).

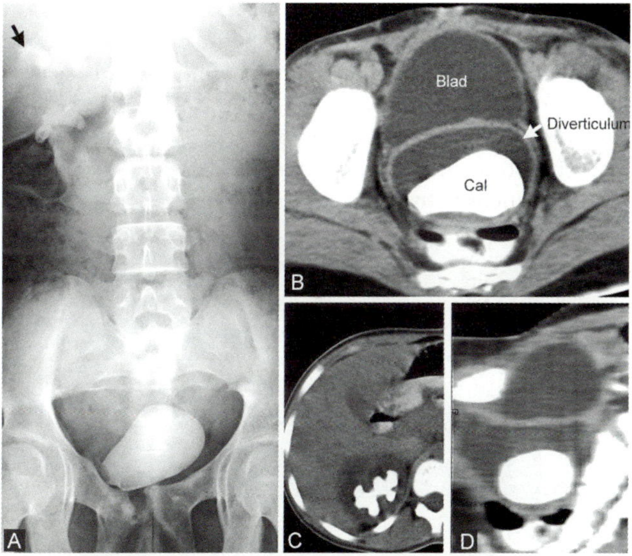

Figures 5.20A to D: A—Plain X-ray abdomen shows multiple staghorn calculi in right kidney and a large calculus in bladder area. B—CT scan demonstrates a large posterior bladder diverticulum with a large calculus. C—The large staghorn calculus in right kidney. D—Sagittal reconstructed CT image shows a posterior diverticulum filled with urine and a large calculus within it.

Bladder Outlet Obstruction

Bladder outlet obstruction can lead to bladder trabeculation, vesicoureteric reflux, hydronephrosis and eventually, to renal parenchymal damage. If no treatment is given, leads to end-stage renal failure. The common clinical manifestation of bladder outlet obstruction is urinary tract infection. Early detection and prevention of deteriorated renal function are important for children with urinary bladder outlet obstruction (Figure 5.21).

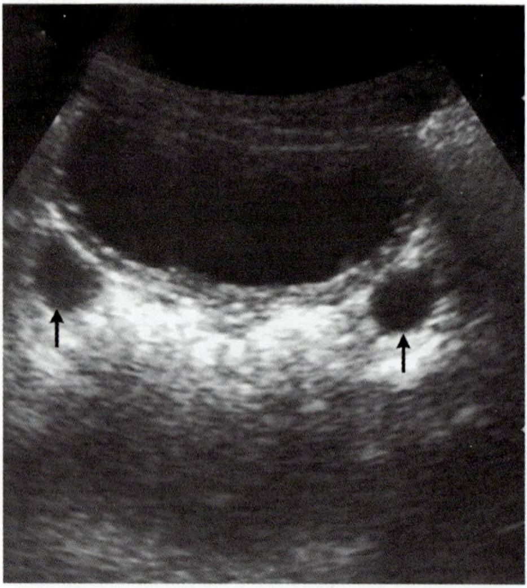

Figure 5.21: Ultrasound shows bilateral hydroureters suggesting bladder outflow obstruction. The bladder wall is thickened.

Retrobladder Abscess

An abscess is a collection of *pus* (*neutrophils*) in a cavity as a result of infection or foreign material. It is a *defensive reaction* of the tissue to prevent the spread of infectious materials to other parts of the body. Treatment of abscess is *surgical* drainage once it has progressed from a harder *serous* inflammation to a softer *pus* stage (Figures 5.22A and B).

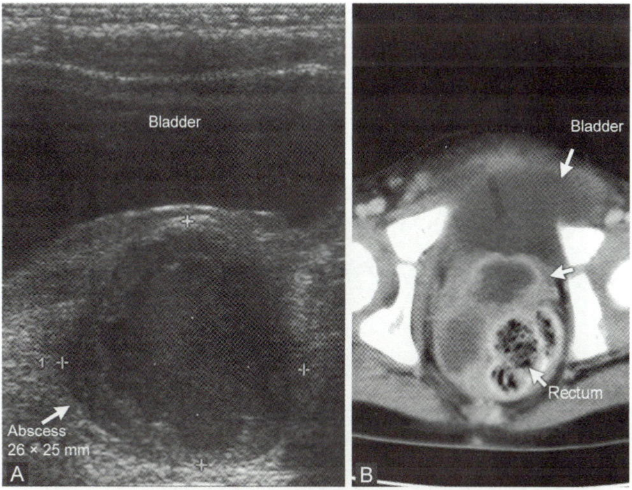

Figures 5.22A and B: Six-year-old child with history of piercing perineal trauma on ultrasound shows a thick walled abscess with internal echos lying posterior to urinary bladder (A). The same is confirmed on CT in which the wall thickness is better appreciated (arrow).

PELVIS

Hydrocele

It is an abnormal collection of serous fluid between the layers of tunica vaginals. It is a common cause of painless scrotal swelling. It can be congenital or acquired. On ultrasound, hydroceles appear as anechoic collection with good acoustic transmission surrounding the anterolateral aspects of the testes. Low level to medium level echoes from fibrin bodies or cholesterol crystal may be found within the hydroceles (Figure 5.23). Large hydrocele may impede testicular venous drainage and cause absence of ante-grade arterial diastolic flow.

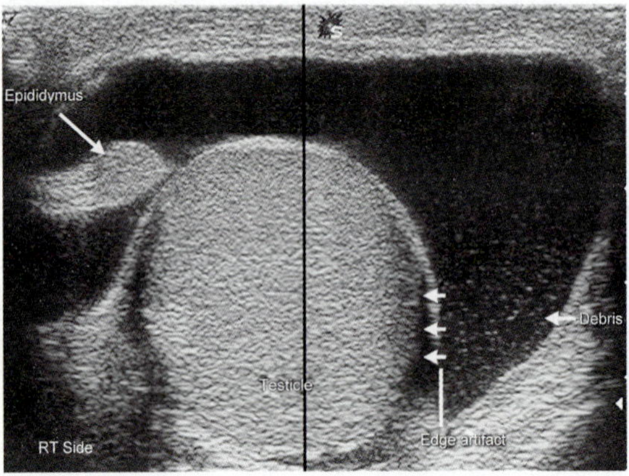

Figure 5.23: USG shows fluid in right tunica vaginalis with internal echos indicating debris. Epididymus is shown by arrow. Three small parallel arrows show edge artifact.

Hypoplastic Uterus

Fifteen-year-old girl referred for primary amenorrhea was found to have a hypoplastic uterus measuring 36x10x13 mm (Figures 5.24A and B). The normal uterus is pear-shaped muscular organ located between the bladder and the rectum. The endometrial cavity is continuous with the cervical canal, and the two openings superiorly lead to the fallopian tubes. The average adolescent uterus is about 7.5 mm long, 5 mm wide and 2.5 mm thick. After menopause, the uterus shrinks to the pre-adolescent size.

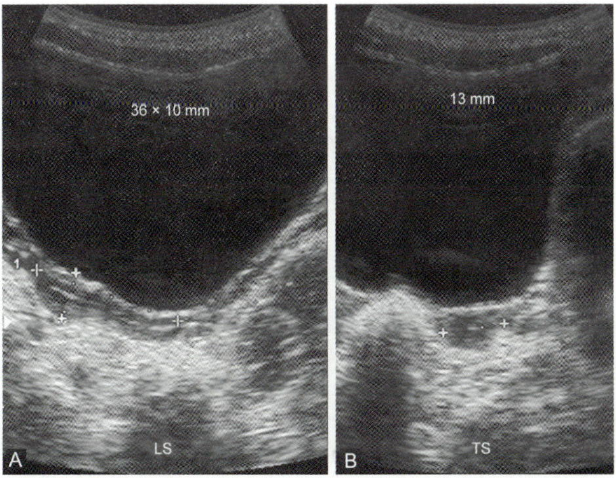

Figures 5.24A and B: Ultrasound shows hypoplastic uterus which measures 36x10 mm in long section (A) and 13 mm thick in cross section (B).

Undescended Testicle (Cryptorchidism)

Right testes is in normal position, left side of scrotal sac is empty. Undescended left testes is lying in proximal end of inguinal canal and is smaller in size. If the testicle cannot be located within the scrotum, it is undescended. An undescended testicle most commonly lies in the inguinal canal or it may lie higher up along the normal line of descent in the abdomen.

If testicles fail to descend by the age of 3 years, it is associated with abnormal development and this is severe at puberty, as a result, undescended testes may be atrophic with poor spermatogenesis.

Ultrasound is regarded as the initial investigation to locate an undescended testicle (Figures 5.25A to C). If not identified on ultrasound, a more extensive search is desired by MRI. CT should be avoided because of radiations. On MR, testicle shows a high signal on T2-weighted and STIR sequences.

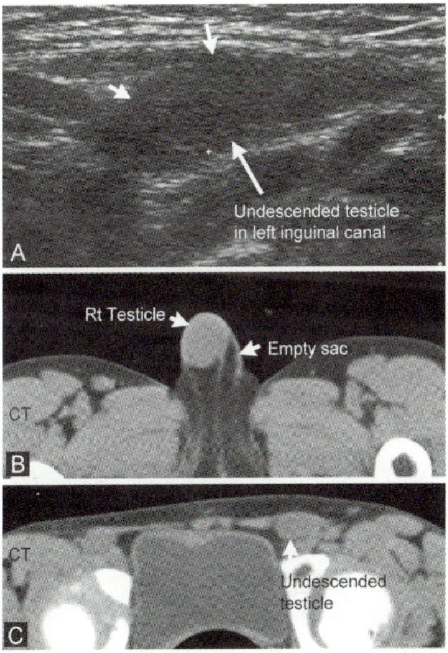

Figures 5.25A to C: A—Left inguinal USG in oblique plane shows the undescended testicle in the inguinal canal (arrows). B—Axial CT image shows right testicle in scrotal sac. The left side of scrotal sac is empty. C—Axial CT image shows undescended testicle in the left inguinal canal.

Chapter Six

Musculoskeletal System

Ashish Ranade
Amol Nade

PREAXIAL AND POSTAXIAL POLYDACTYLY

Polydactyly may be preaxial (radial) or postaxial (ulnar). It may range from an ossicle to complete duplication of fingers or toes. On occasion the hand may be duplicated. When present, should search for an associated syndrome. Syndactyly may be associated with polydactyly. Postaxial polydactyly is more frequent and often seen as fifth digit duplications in hands or feet (Figures 6.1A to D).

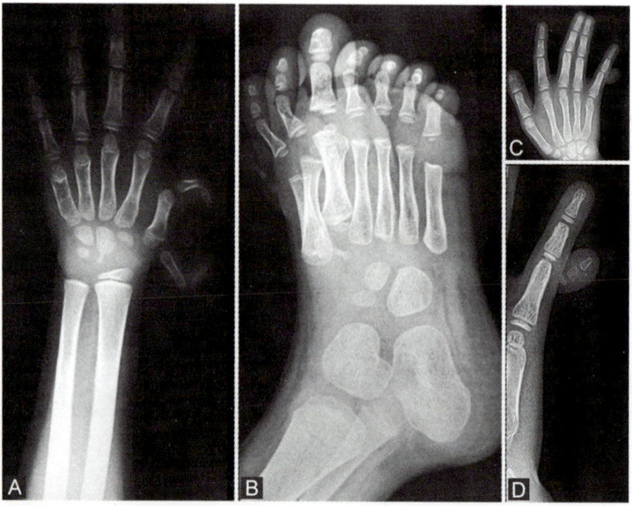

Figures 6.1A to D: A—AP radiograph of hand shows pre-axial (radial) polydactyly in a six-year-old female. B—Oblique radiograph of foot shows pre-axial polydactyly in 14-year-old male. C—shows post-axial (ulnar) polydactyly. D—is magnified view of C.

ECTRODACTYLY ECTODERMAL DYSPLASIA CLEFT LIP (EEC) SYNDROME

Ectrodactyly Ectodermal Dysplasia Cleft Lip (EEC) syndrome is a uncommon condition with multiple congenital anomalies with normal intelligence characterized by ectodermal dysplasia, clefting of hands, feet, lip and palate. It is an autosomal dominant syndrome. Management of the cases requires a multidisciplinary approach. Early diagnosis allows precise counseling of parents with reassurance of normal intelligence.

Examination of the baby revealed ectrodactyly (splitting of hands and feet), ectodermal dysplasia, cleft lip and palate, sparse scalp hairs and eyebrows and absence of eye lashes. These abnormalities constitute the EEC syndrome (Figures 6.2A to E)

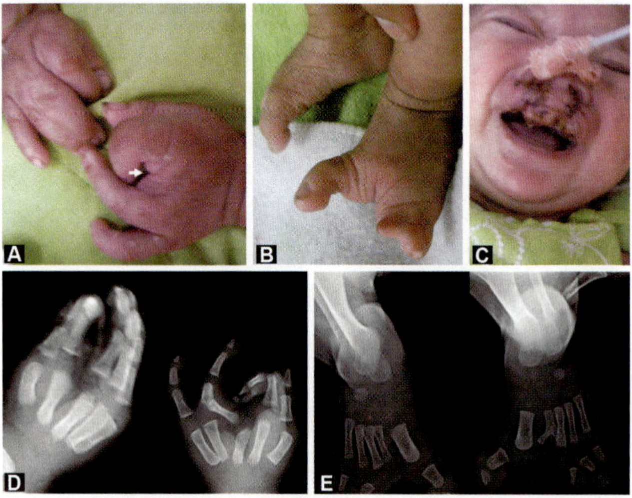

Figures 6.2A to E: Both hands have claw like appearance due to cone shaped defect (arrow). Soft tissue fusion of the middle and ring finger of the right hand and index and middle finger of the left hand is seen (A). Both feet show claw like appearance due to soft tissue fusion of the 3rd, 4th and 5th toes (B). Surgery has been performed for cleft lip (C). X-ray hands (D) show a cone-shaped defect. There is absence of middle and distal phalanges of middle finger on the left side. X-ray feet (E) show cone shaped defect due to absence of 2nd toe on either side. Syndactyly of the metatarsals of the left foot is seen. There is absence of middle and distal phalanges of 3rd, 4th and 5th toes on either side.

MADELUNG'S DEFORMITY

Madelung's deformity is common in girls and is generally bilateral and presents during adolescence. The defective development of the inner third of the epiphysis of the lower end of the radius results in bowing of radial shaft thus increasing the interosseous space. The lower end of ulna is subluxed backward. The hand projects forward at the wrist joint to produce a bayonet-like appearance in a lateral projection (Figure 6.3).

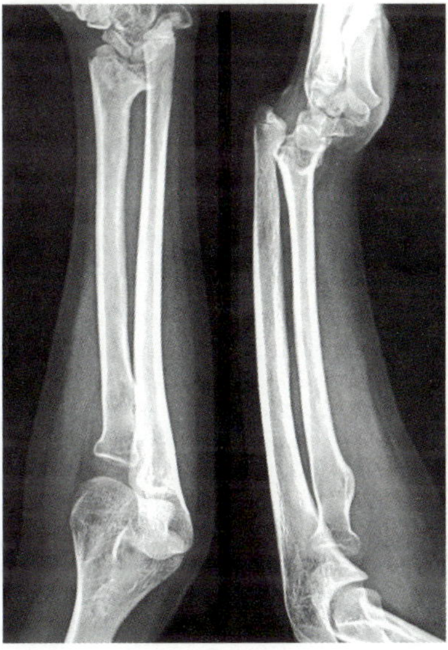

Figure 6.3: Madelung's deformity of right wrist in a 13-year-old female

CONGENITAL HIP DISLOCATION

Congenital hip dislocation is a very important condition as treatment depends upon early recognition. Females are more commonly affected (F>M, 5:1). Dislocation is usually unilateral (L>R, 11:1), both hips may be involved. Ultrasound is now the accepted method of primary investigation of suspected developmental dysplasia of the hip (Figure 6.4).

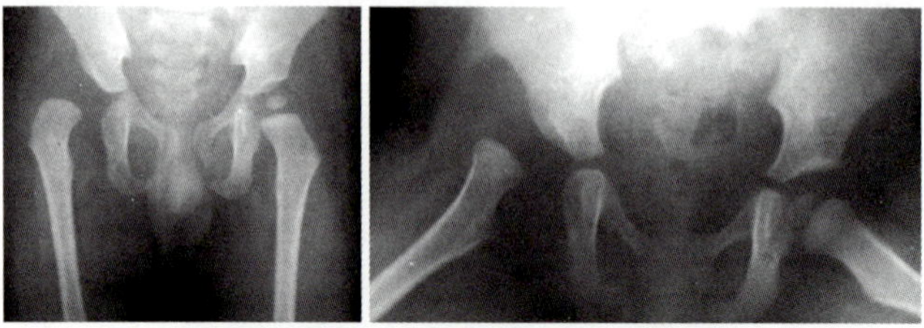

Figure 6.4: AP and frog pelvis radiographs shows congenital hip dislocation in a 3-year-old male.

OSTEONECROSIS OF HIP (LEGG-CALVE-PERTHES DISEASE)

Perthes is a self-limiting disease seen between 3 to 12 years of age, more common in boys. Patient presents with a limp. The underlying pathology is vascular occlusive episodes of femoral head; the ossific nucleus of the epiphysis suffers necrosis causing growth arrest. Cartilage overlying the femoral head thickens followed by remodeling. Plain radiographs show growth retardation with reduced size of capital femoral epiphysis, subchondral fissuring and fractures and increased density of ossific nucleus. The amount of subchondral fissuring of the femoral head during the initial stages is thought to have prognostic predictive value, the prognosis is poor when associated with more than 50% subchondral fissuring (Figures 6.9A and B).

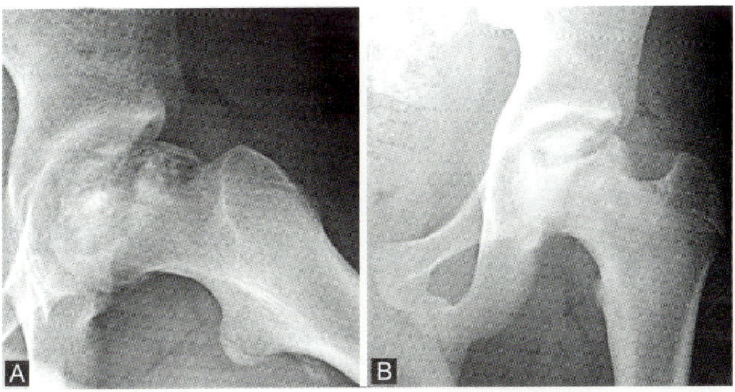

Figures 6.9A and B: A—X-ray left hip shows reduced size and subchondral fissuring of capital femoral epiphysis. B—shows reduced size, fissuring, fragmentation and increased density of capital femoral epiphysis.

OSTEOID OSTEOMA

Osteoid osteoma is a benign lesion frequently found in the appendicular skeleton. The tumors produce excess bone and secrete pain-causing prostaglandins, resulting in intense pain especially at night. A 17-year-old male presented with pain and tenderness in left thigh region since 4 months. Radiograph shows sclerosis and cortical thickening due to subperiosteal bone formation. The radiolucent nidus is questionably visualized. The location of the nidus, intranidal calcification, sclerosis, mature periosteal bone formation and location of original cortex is precisely demonstrated by CT. MRI also clearly showed the partially calcified nidus and associated cortical thickening. In addition, MR images revealed mild marrow and soft tissue edema in the vicinity of the nidus, which is not demonstrated by CT (Figures 6.10A to E).

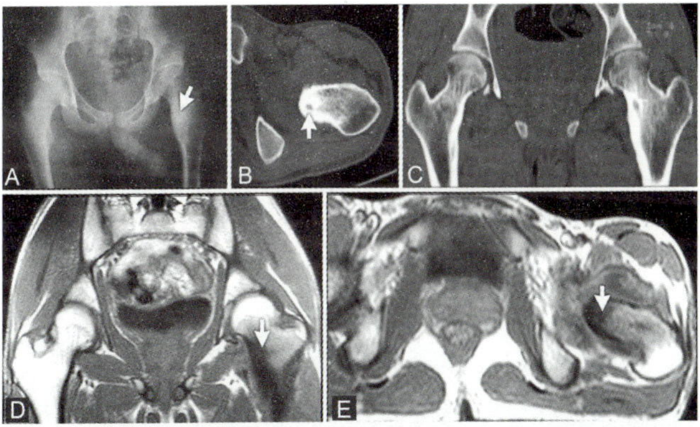

Figures 6.10A to E: Plain radiograph of 17-year-old male shows (A) an ill-defined region of increased cortical thickness (arrow) and CT axial (B) and coronal reformatted (C) reveals the presence of small well defined calcified nidus and dense cortical thickening near lesser trochanter. MRI coronal (D) and axial (E) reveals hypointense cortical thickening along lesser trochanter with well defined small hypointense lesion adjacent to it (arrow).

RICKETS

Vitamin D deficiency causes rickets due to failure of mineralization of bone and cartilage. The radiological findings at the epiphyseal plate reveal the changed pathophysiology. The normal maturation and mineralization of cartilage cells becomes disrupted. The plain radiograph features show osteopenia, widening of growth plate strikingly seen in long bones, cupping of metaphysis (Figures 6.11A to D), metaphyseal bands indicative of ill-defined zone of provisional calcification, bowing deformities of bones especially the lower limbs and rachitic rosary (enlargement of costochondral junction).

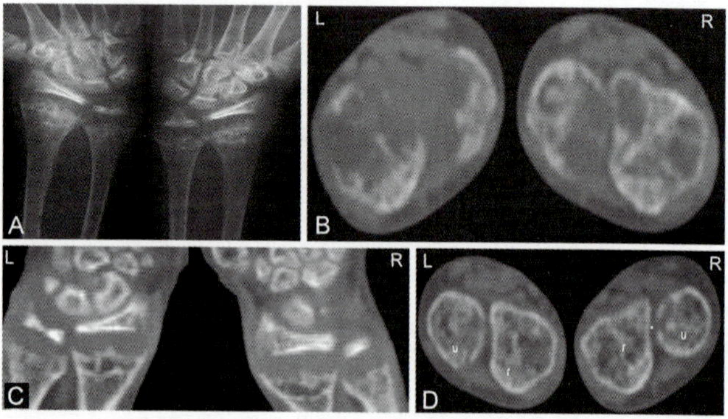

Figures 6.11A to D: A—X-ray of both wrists and hands shows osteomalacia with widening of growth plate, splaying and cupping of distal metaphysis of radius and ulna with irregular metaphyseal margins. CT axial and coronal reconstructed images confirm the X-ray findings of defective mineralization of osteoid tissue in cortical and cancellous bone (B to D). These are features of rickets.

CHRONIC OSTEOMYELITIS

Chronic osteomyelitis results from failure to eliminate the acute or subacute osteomyelitis, or from local spread of soft tissue infection, complication of compound fractures, or following surgery. Radiographs show bone destruction and focal cortical thickening due to periosteal new bone formation, cortical defects and sequestrum with modeling deformities and soft tissue irregularities can also be seen (Figure 6.12). The sequelae include: (a) Growth plate destruction leading to limb length discrepancy, (b) Chronically discharging, (c) Extensive bone destruction with modeling deformity, (d) Avascular necrosis, (e) Pathological fractures, and (f) Premature osteoarthritis.

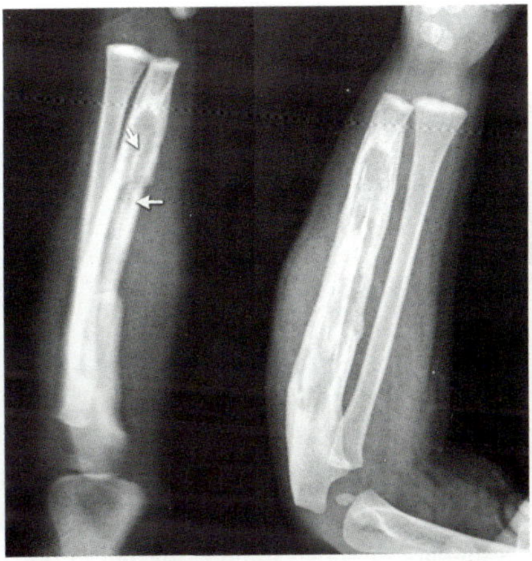

Figure 6.12: X-ray left forearm of a three-year-old male with chronic osteomyelitis, ulna shows cortical thickening, bone destruction and sequestrum formation (arrow).

SEPTIC ARTHRITIS

Infectious arthritis affects children and hip joint is a common site to be involved. Spread of infection may be hematogeous, local trauma, neighboring osteomyelitis or adjoining soft tissue infection. Streptococcus Group is frequently implicated. The avascular joint cartilage gets infected through the highly vascular synovial membrane causing edema and effusion, the obliteration of cartilage leads to reduction of joint space and destroys the articular cartilage. Followed by immobilization due to pain leads to osteoporosis and destruction leading to subluxations or dislocations. Other sequelae are fibrous ankylosis and deformity. Initially, radiographs may show joint space widening with soft tissue swelling. Later osteoporosis, loss of joint space, marginal and central erosion of articular cortex is seen (Figure 6.13).

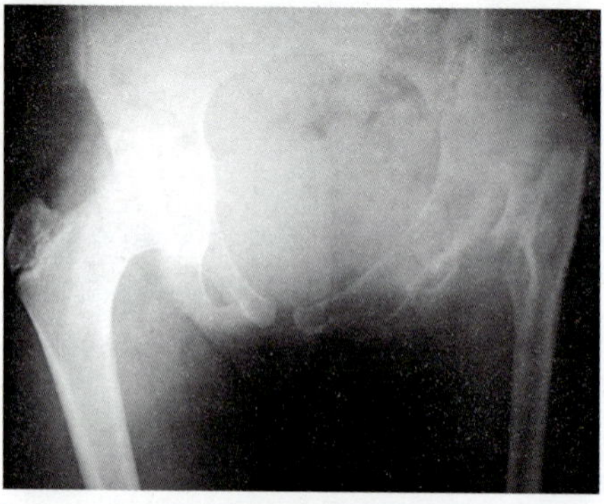

Figure 6.13: Sequelae in septic arthritis left hip in an eight-year-old female in the form of destruction of left femoral head which is displaced superiorly with development of pseudoarthrosis.

OSTEOCHONDROMA RIB

Osteochondroma or exostosis is benign bony excrescence with a cartilage cap. It may be solitary or multiple (It has been estimated that rib osteochondromas arise in almost 50% of patients with multiple hereditary exostoses). The rib exostoses that project externally are palpable on the chest wall. Osteochondromas can mimic pulmonary nodules. CT is most helpful in determining the nature of these bone growths (Figure 6.14).

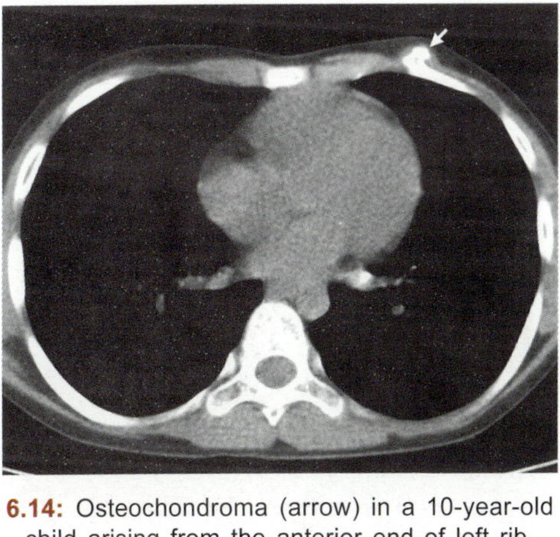

Figure 6.14: Osteochondroma (arrow) in a 10-year-old female child arising from the anterior end of left rib.

Chapter
Seven

PET-CT and MR-PET

Sikandar Shaikh

PET-CT

Positron emission tomography—computed tomography (PET-CT) has transformed the field of medical diagnosis, PET alone lacked anatomic localization and CT lacked functional aspect of imaging. PET-CT has the advantages of both modalities, i.e. PET and CT. Patient is subjected to both the modalities in the same session and images are acquired. The system combines the images into superimposed images. In this way, functional imaging obtained by PET, which depicts the distribution of metabolic or biochemical activity in the body is aligned to the anatomic image obtained by CT.

PET-CT is used for early diagnosis of malignant diseases, its staging and follow-up, surgical planning and radiation therapy and response to treatment. It determines the location and extent of cancer indicating spread to other areas of the body such as lymph nodes, liver, bones or brain in the form of metastatic disease. It distinguishes between malignant and benign tumors and recurrent cancer from scar tissue or fibrosis.

PET-CT is also used to study brain function in epilepsy, diagnosing Alzheimer's disease and other types of dementia, evaluating viability of heart muscle and study of coronary artery disease.

2-Deoxy-2-(18f), fluoro-deoxy-glucose or 18F-FDG, is a radioactive form of glucose and is the most common radiopharmaceutical used in PET. 18F-FDG has a half-life of approximately 110 minutes, so it is quickly expelled from the body. It is produced by cyclotron. Other radioisotope-positron emitters which can be used are fluorine-18, carbon-11, nitrogen-13 and oxygen-15, having much shorter half lifes.

Patient is kept fasting for atleast 4 hours prior to scan. 10 mCi (370 MBq) of 18F-FDG is injected and imaging is done after one hour. Normal PET image shows more uptake in brain and cardiac muscles where there is increased metabolism. Pelvicalyceal system and urinary bladder show high uptake due to excretion.

Standardized uptake value (SUV) enables comparison within and between different patients and diseases.

$$\text{SUV} = \frac{\text{Radionuclide distribution in region of interest}}{\text{Radionuclide dose injected/Patient's weight in kg}}$$

Sr. No.	*Region*	*SUV*
1.	Soft tissue	0.6–0.8
2.	Liver	2.2–2.5
3.	Kidneys	3.3–3.5
4.	Neoplasm	5.0–20.0

PET-CT Gantry

First the patient is put through CT gantry and CT scan is done and patient is shifted further into the PET gantry. Thus first the CT images are acquired followed by PET images and these images are then fused by software resulting in PET-CT images (Figure 7.1).

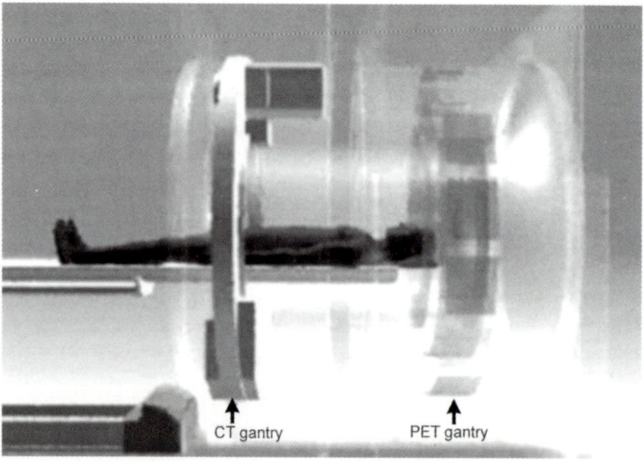

Figure 7.1: PET-CT gantry

Cyclotron

Cyclotron is the equipment with the help of which 18F-FDG glucose is prepared in 5 hours. FDG glucose is tagged to fluorine molecule resulting in 18F-FDG glucose molecule used for PET imaging (Figure 7.2).

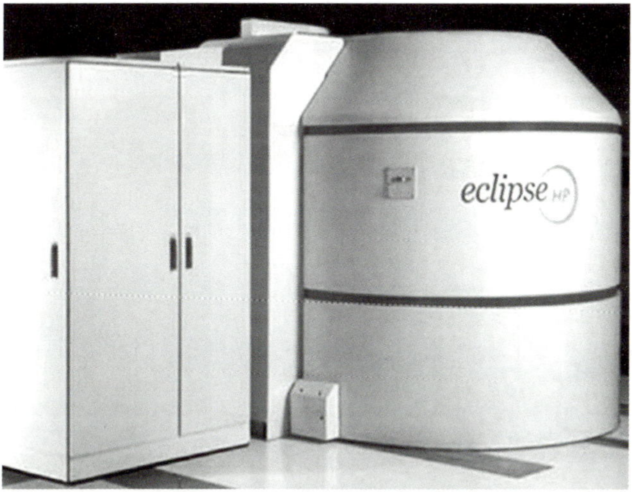

Figure 7.2: Cyclotron

MEDIASTINAL LYMPHOMA

A fourteen-year-old boy presented with gradually increasing breathlessness and vague chest pain.

X-ray showed superior mediastinal widening. CT chest revealed an anterior mediastinal mass (arrow) infiltrating the anterior mediastinal structures. Confirmed as lymphoma. PET-CT was done for staging which did not reveal any distant metastases (Figure 7.3).

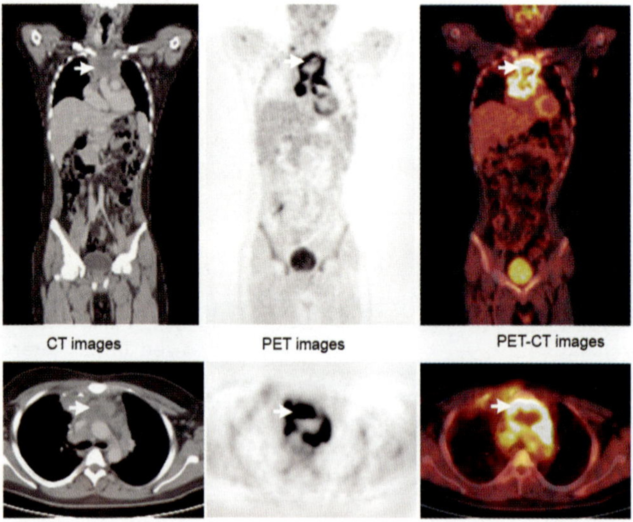

Figure 7.3

RESTAGING OF MEDULLOBLASTOMA AFTER SURGERY (FIGURE 7.4)

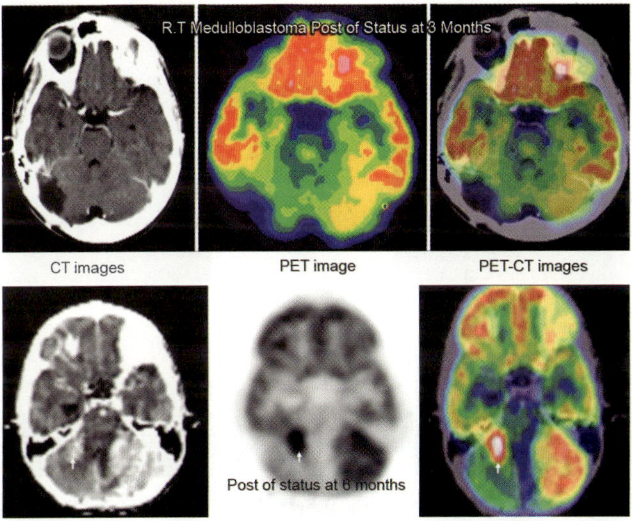

Figure 7.4: A five-year old male child presented with imbalance on walking with headache on and off. CT showed large heterogeneously enhancing lesion in right cerebellum. Surgical excision of the mass carried out. Histopathologically confirmed it as medulloblastoma. Postoperative PET-CT brain was done showed no residual lesion. Three months after surgery patient had vague headache. PET-CT was repeated and it did not show any residual lesion or recurrence. Symptoms increased and PET-CT was again performed at 6 months after surgery showed recurrence of lesion in right cerebellum (arrows).

NASOPHARYNGEAL SQUAMOUS CELL CARCINOMA (FIGURE 7.5)

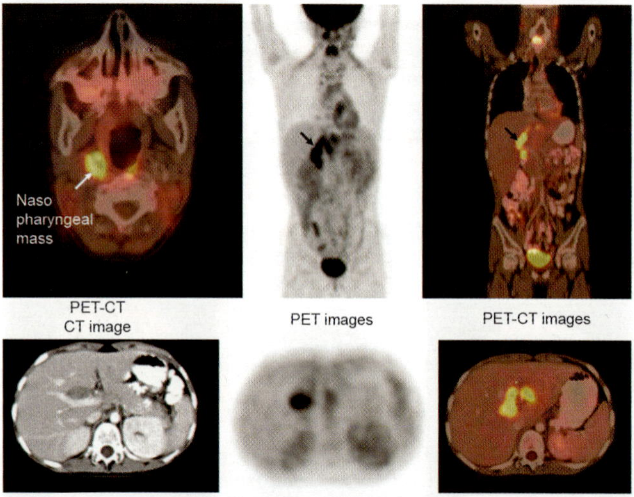

Figure 7.5: A 13-year-old boy presented with gradually increasing neck pain of one month duration. On CT scan revealed a right nasopharyngeal mass (white arrow) confirmed as squamous cell carcinoma. Whole body PET-CT showed liver metastases (black arrow). Thyroid shows diffuse nonspecific uptake.

PERICARDIAL ANGIOSARCOMA (FIGURE 7.6)

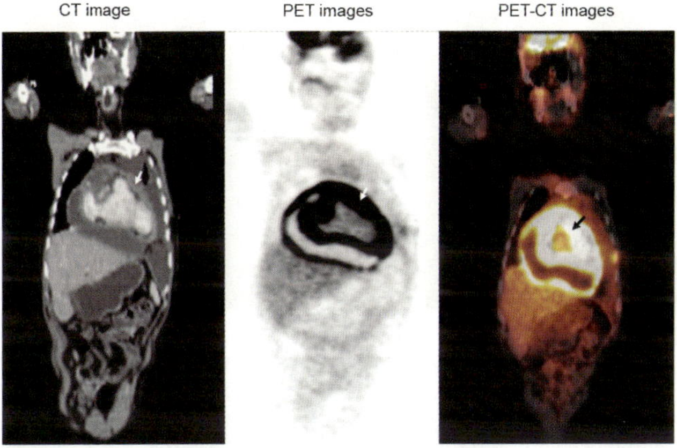

Figure 7.6: A 15-year-old female presented with progressive breathlessness and constitutional symptoms. X-ray chest revealed significant cardiomegaly. CT chest showed pericardial thickening (arrow) with pericardial effusion. Pericardial fluid was aspirated and histopathologically confirmed as pericardial angiosarcoma. PET-CT for staging showed only local disease.

WILMS' TUMOR (FIGURE 7.7)

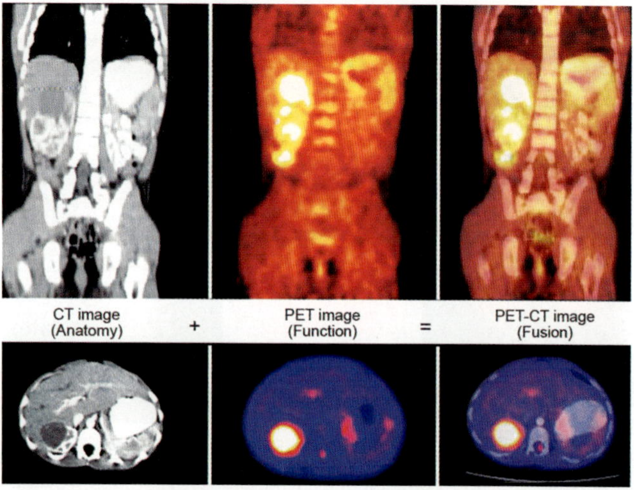

Figure 7.7: An 8-year-old male presented with urinary symptoms. Limited PET-CT abdomen done to avoid more radiation. CT shows mass in upper pole of right kidney. PET image shows increased uptake but can be mistaken for pelvicalyceal system, so CT scan is mandatory in renal pathologies. PET-CT image shows increased uptake with void in central area corresponding to the necrosis on CT.

MR-PET

Prototypes of integrated MR systems (Figure 7.8) that can produce simultaneous, integrated images of the brain (Figure 7.9) are currently under development and not commercially available. MRI gives structural details and provides high soft tissue resolution images whereas positron emission tomography (PET) uses a radioactive tracer in the body to obtain functional information of a particular organ or system, locate metastasis, recurrence of tumors and help in determining the effectiveness of treatment in malignant diseases. However, PET gives molecular detail but fails to give anatomical information. The combined capability of MR-PET has been developed while PET evaluates the metabolic aspects and MRI gives high resolution anatomical information.

MR-PET gains over PET-CT are that MR-PET provides excellent soft tissue image and the patient is not exposed to radiations. PET-MRI can differentiate tumor recurrence from fibrosis following radiotherapy.

MR-PET is a modality with tremendous potential for combining structure and function. The images of both MR-PET are useful to diagnose intricate cases, planning and treatment and follow up. In addition to imaging tumors and conducting functional studies, MR-PET may also lead to increased understanding of diseases like Alzheimer's, Parkinson's, stroke, depression, and schizophrenia, and could even help refine surgery. MR-PET once made available will revolutionize the field of medicine on treatment and follow up of cases.

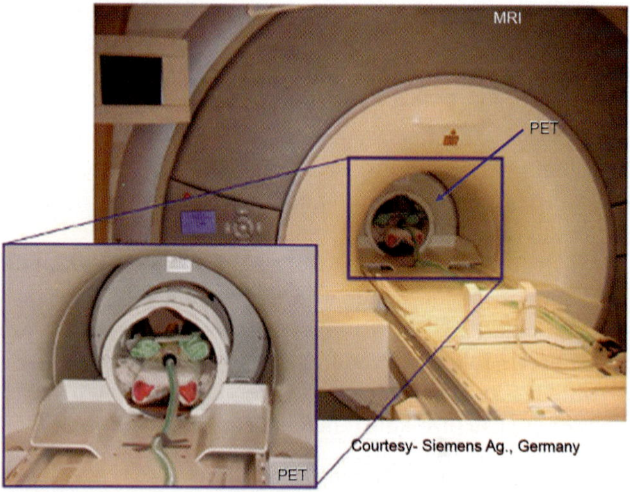

Figure 7.8: MR-PET equipment, in this each scan occurs without repositioning the patient.

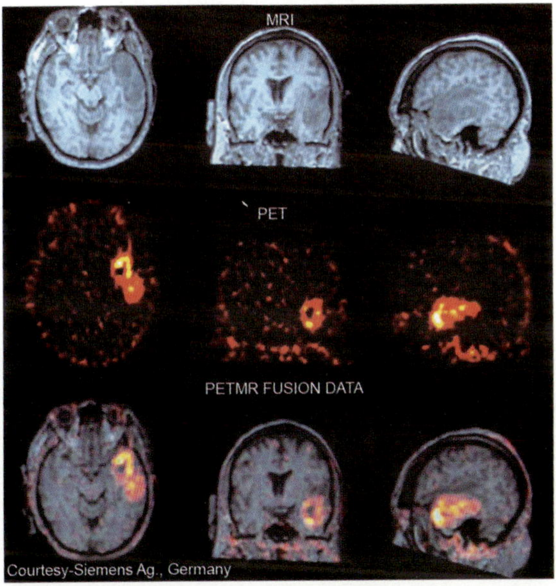

Figure 7.9: MR, PET and Fusion images demonstrates the glioma proliferation.

CHAPTER
Eight

Miscellaneous Cluster

Hariqbal Singh

DIVERSE CASES

Agnathia

Agnathia or otocephaly, is characterized by microstomia (small mouth), aglossia (absence of the tongue), agnathia (absence of the lower jaw) and ear abnormalities. Most babies who have this condition do not survive. Polyhydramnios is frequently found with agnathia. Both genetic and environmental factors have an impact on this condition. Most reported cases have been sporadic. The diagnosis can sometimes be made on ultrasound but is difficult (Figures 8.1A to D).

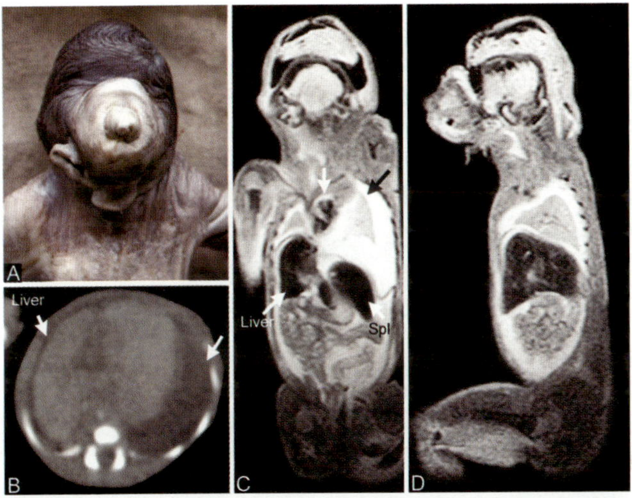

Figures 8.1A to D: A—24 weeks' aborted fetus shows absence of the opening of the mouth, lower jaw and left ear with snout like nose. CT scan (B) and MRI T2WI (C), shows presence of pleural fluid (black arrow), ascites (white arrow) and pericardial effusion (block arrow). Spleen is large. Subscalp air seen in C and D is secondary to intervention.

Lymph Nodes

Most lymph nodes on ultrasound appear ovoid in shape and are variable in size, vary in echogenicity although a few of them are homogeneous depending on the degree of central lipomatosis. The center of the node is echogenic and the periphery is hypoechoic. Not all enlarged nodes are malignant and not all malignant nodes are enlarged. Normally 1 to 3 mm central artery is present at the hilum of lymph node. In malignant involvement this central artery is not seen because it is infiltrated and destroyed (Figures 8.2A and B).

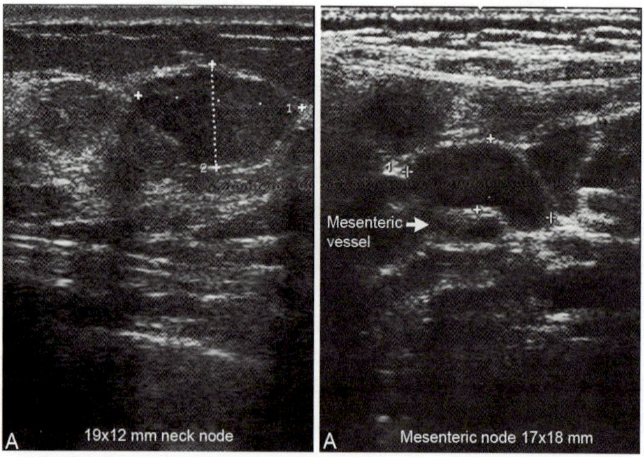

Figures 8.2A and B: Ultrasound shows neck (A) and mesenteric (B) lymph modes.

Fetus in Fetu

Fetus in fetu is a rare clinical entity and diagnosis can be accurately made by CT imaging. The demonstration of spinal elements is the most definite of this condition to differentiate from a teratoma (Figures 8.3A to D).

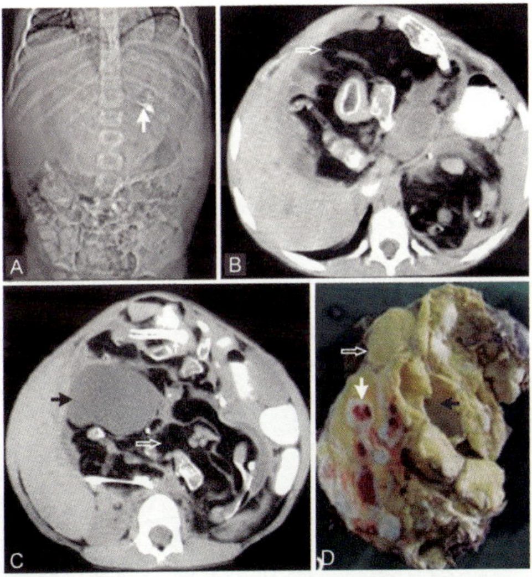

Figures 8.3A to D: A five-year-old male presented with a palpable mass in upper abdomen since birth. CT images revealed a large heterogeneous density mass lesion in the peritoneal cavity displacing the normal structures. The mass showed solid, cystic (black arrow), fatty (block arrow) and osseous (white arrow) components. Few well formed tubular bones and joints are seen. The fat plane between the lesion and adjacent abdominal structures is well-defined. Complete surgical excision of the lesion was performed and the diagnosis was confirmed on histopathology.

Jeune's Syndrome

Jeune's syndrome is a rare genetic disorder, an autosomal recessive dysplasia also known as asphyxiating thoracic dystrophy. It is characterized by short limbs, narrow rigid and abnormally small thoracic cage (Figures 8.4A to C) with reduced lung capacity. Ribs are short and have irregular and bulbous costochondral junctions. They have reduced thoracic mobility and predominant abdominal breathing. Individuals with Jeune's syndrome may also develop high blood pressure from renal disease.

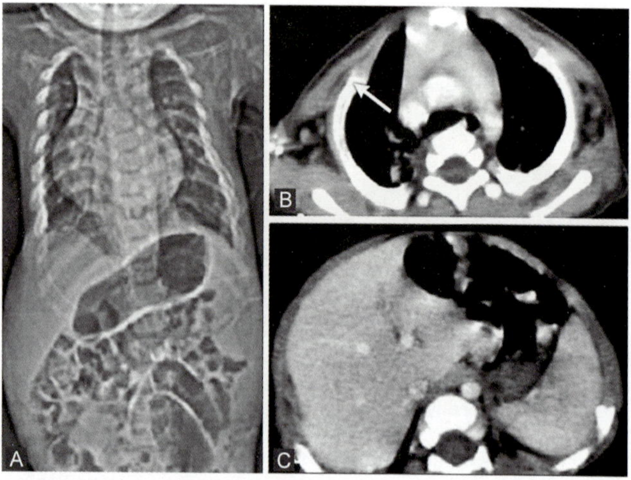

Figures 8.4A to C: Chest is long, narrow and small with reduced lung capacity. Thoracic diameter is significantly less as compared to abdomen.

CT GUIDED PRECISION BIOPSY

CT guided precision robotic assistance biopsy with automated planner. Automated planning reduces the number of needle passes, time spent and number of check scans which leads to significant reduction to patient's radiation dosage.

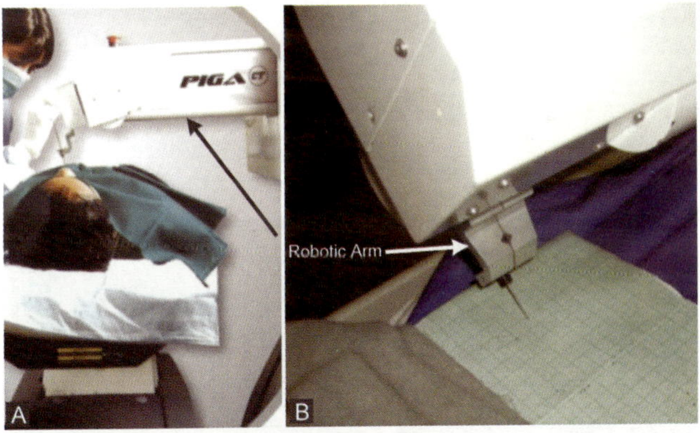

Figures 8.5A and (B): A—PIGA^{CT}CT guided precision robotic assistance biopsy automated planner. B—Magnified view of the robotic arm with biopsy needle.

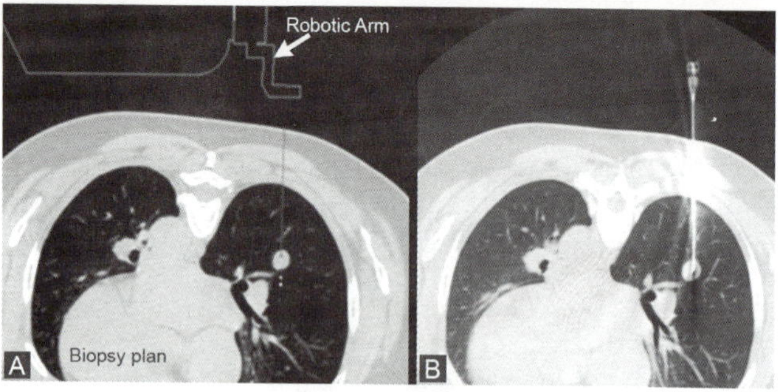

Figures 8.6A and B: A—Plan for posterior straight approach biopsy (red line) for a 12 mm nodule in right lung. B—Check scan shows precise positioning of needle in the nodule.

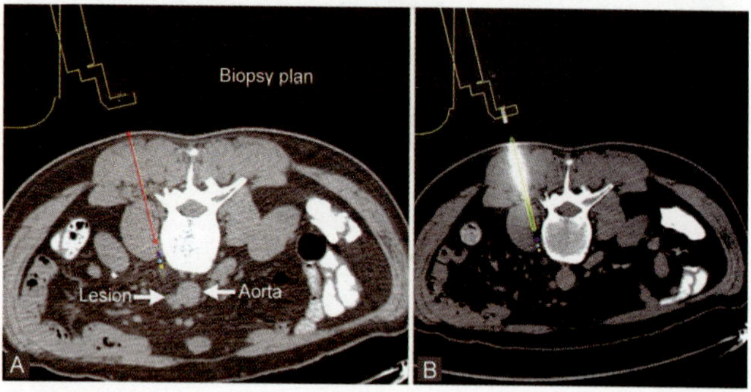

Figures 8.7A and B: A—Posterior approach biopsy plan for a 9 mm left para-aortic lymph node. B—The needle held in robotic arm is in the process of moving into the left para-aortic lymph node.

MULTIPLE EPIPHYSEAL DYSPLASIA

It is characterized by an abnormality of mucopolysaccharoid and glycoprotein metabolism and develops in early childhood. Radiographs show delayed ossification and delayed mineralization of the epiphysis of long bones which are fragmented small and flattened, loose bodies may also occur in joints (Figure 6.5). Metaphyseal irregularity is seen in tubular bones, when spine is involved there is irregularity of vertebral end plates.

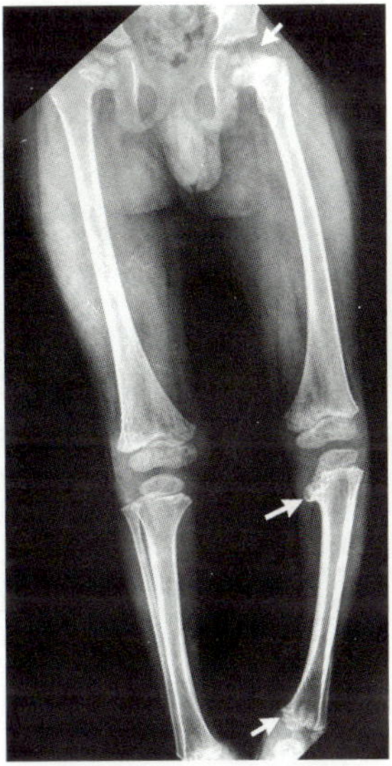

Figure 6.5: A 5-year-old male with multiple epiphyseal dysplasia shows bilateral involvement of long bones of lower limbs.

MACRODYSTROPHIA LIPOMATOSA

Macrodystrophia lipomatosa is a congenital local gigantism of the hand and foot, characterized by proliferation of all mesenchymal components, particularly fibroadipose tissue (Figures 6.6A to C and 6.7A and B). Macrodystrophia lipomatosa comes to clinical attention because of cosmetic reasons, mechanical problems secondary to degenerative joint disease or development of neurovascular compression.

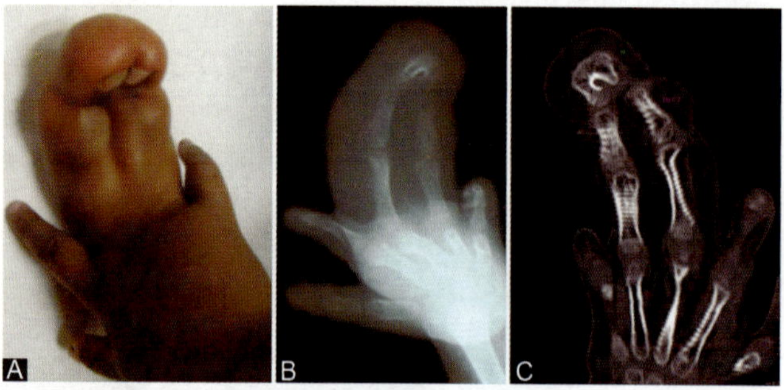

Figures 6.6A to C: A—Clinical photograph of right hand shows enlarged, fused ring and middle finger. Plain radiograph (B) and coronal reformatted CT (C) shows soft tissue swelling and proliferation of fat on palmar aspect of the ring and middle fingers, along with dorsal angulation and syndactyly.

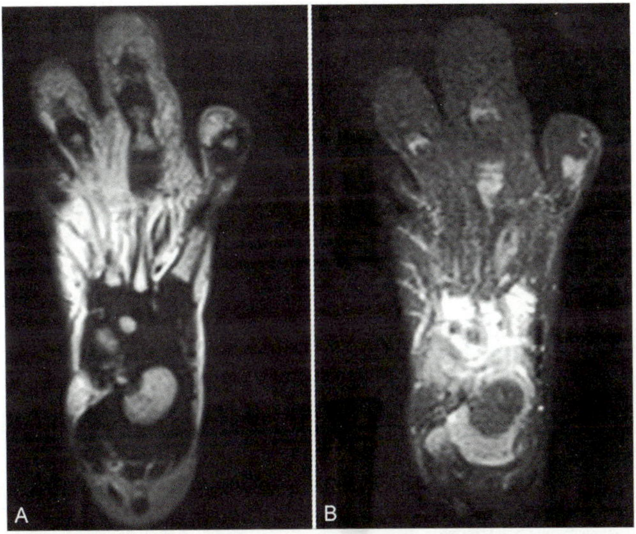

Figures 6.7A and B: T1 Coronal MRI (A) reveals proliferation of fatty tissue on plantar aspect of the second and third toes of right foot with signal intensity similar to that of subcutaneous fat as seen by fat suppressed STIR coronal image (B).

HOLT-ORAM SYNDROME

Holt-Oram syndrome is an inherited disorder that causes abnormalities of the hands, arms, spine and heart. Occurs approximately in one in every 100,000 and affects both sexes equally.

It falls into two groups: A—Defects in arm and hand bones involving one or both sides of the body. Most commonly the defects are in the carpal bones and thumb. The thumb may be malformed or missing. In severe cases the arms may be very short such that the hands are attached close to the body (phocomelia). B—Heart abnormalities. Three-fourth of cases with Holt-Oram syndrome have heart abnormality. It may be abnormal rhythms, *atrial* or *ventricular septal defect* (Figures 6.8A to D).

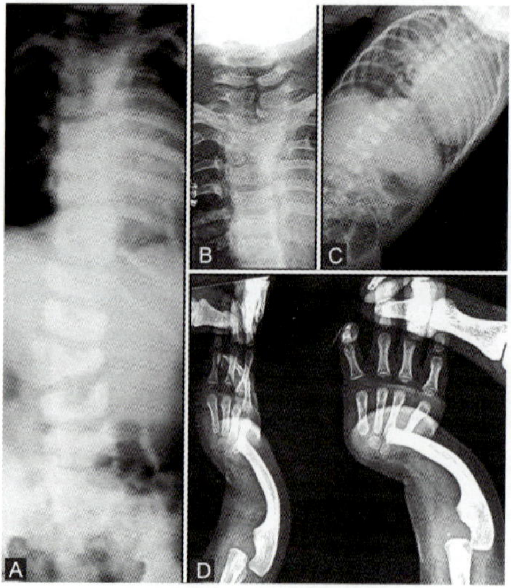

Figures 6.8A to D: A and B—X-rays spine show multiple spinal anomalies. C—shows congenital heart disease. D—shows absence of radius. All these are features of Holt-Oram syndrome.

SPOTTERS

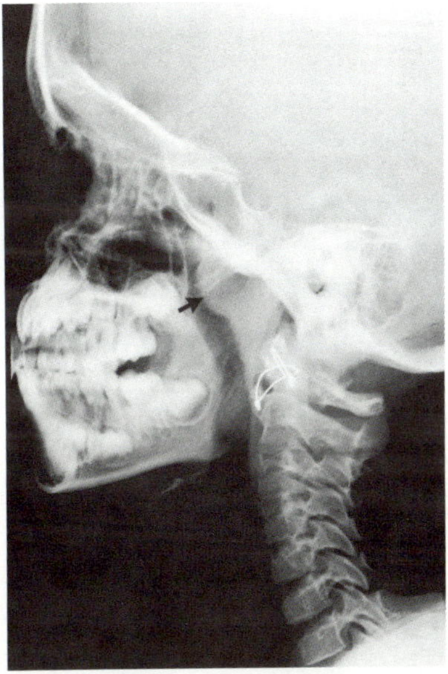

Figure 8.8: Enlarged adenoid in a seven-year-old child.

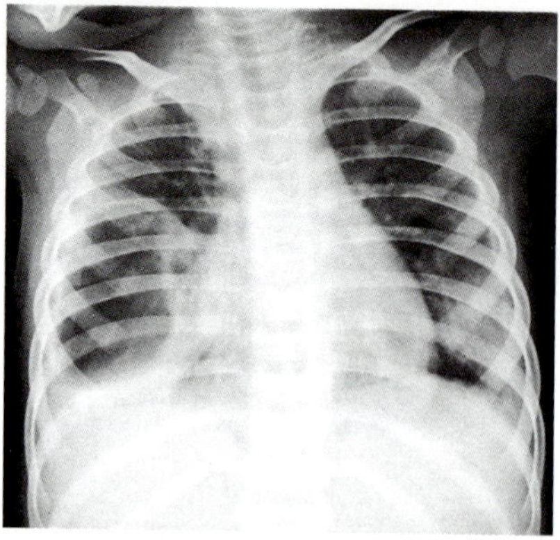

Figure 8.9: X-ray chest of one-year-old child with right lung abscess, air fluid level is seen. Left lung shows left lower zone consolidation.

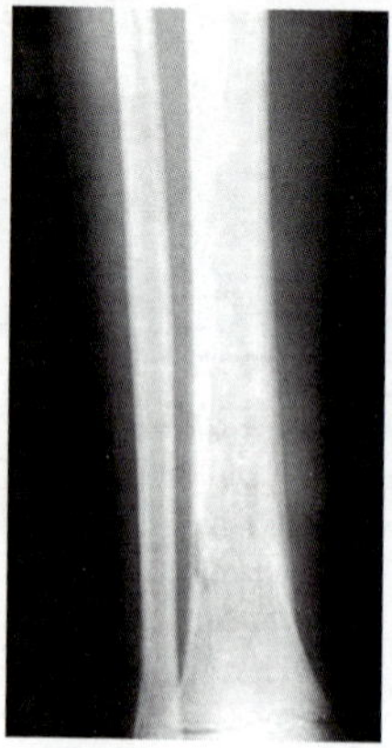

Figure 8.10: X-ray leg shows osteomyelitis of tibia seen as periosteal reaction.

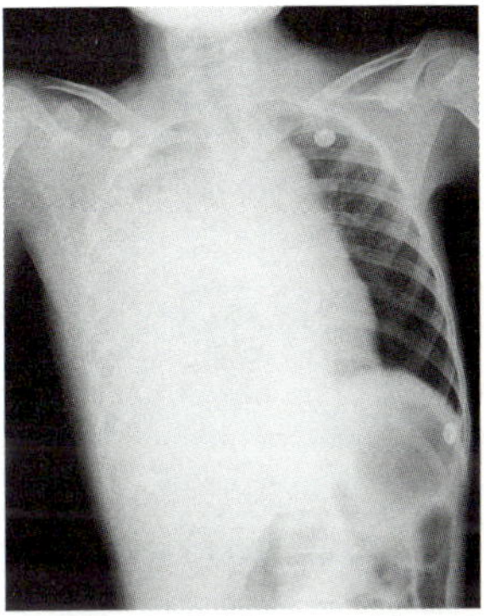

Figure 8.11: X-ray chest of 12-year-old male shows pleural effusion with collapse consolidation of right lung.

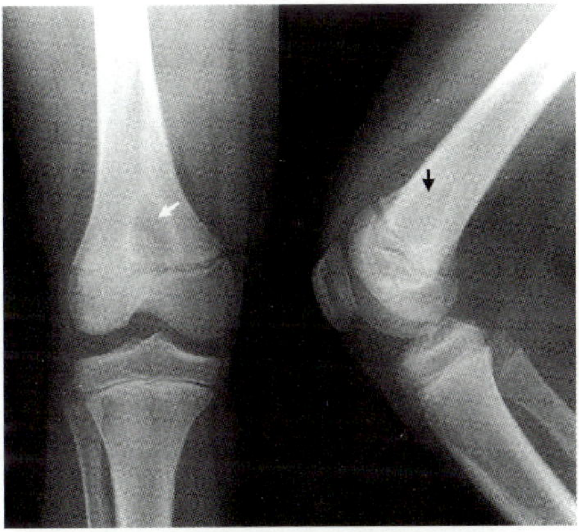

Figure 8.12: X-ray knee shows Brodie's abscess at distal end tibia extending into the epiphyseal line.

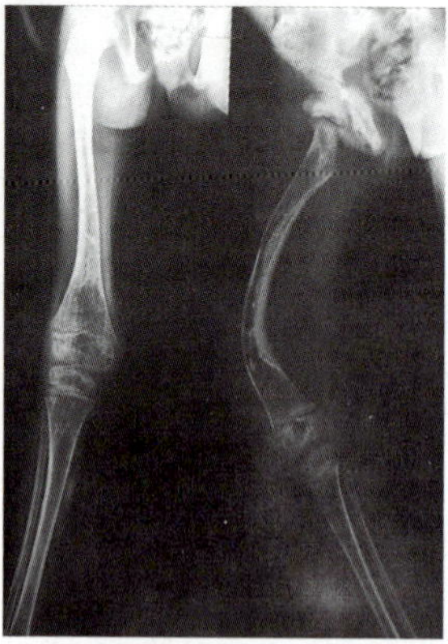

Figure 8.13: AP and lateral radiographs show valgus procurvatum deformity of right femur in a seven-year-old female child with rickets.

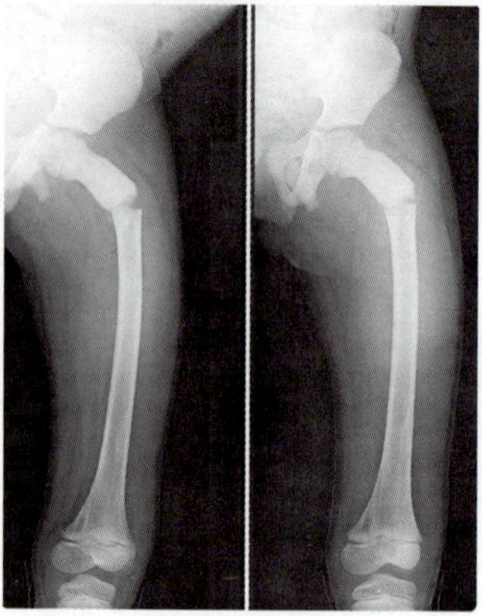

Figure 8.14: X-ray thigh shows fibrous dysplasia with pathological fracture of left femur.

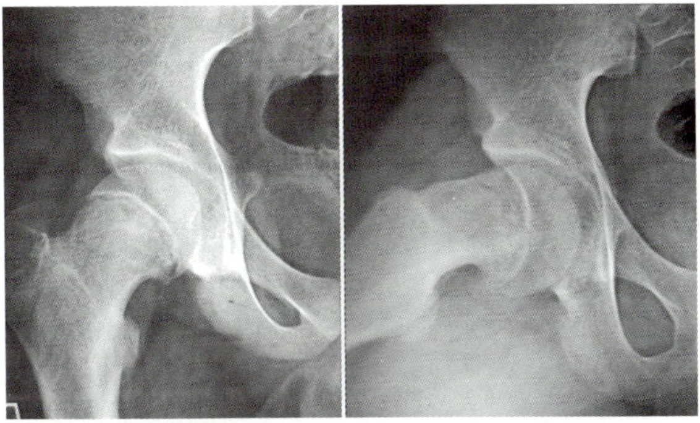

Figure 8.15: AP and frog views of pelvis radiographs show slipped capital femoral epiphysis in a 14-year-old male.

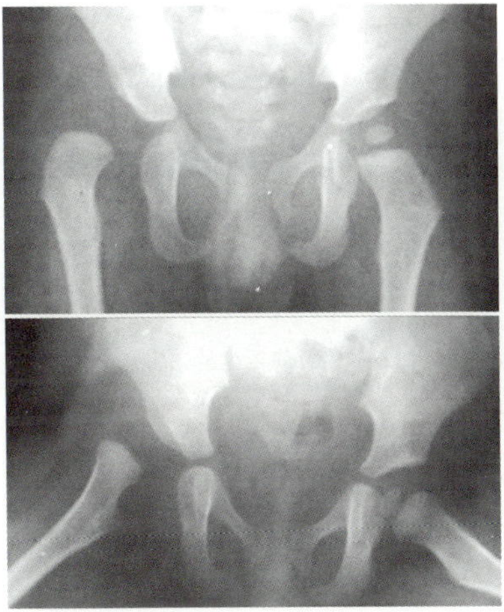

Figure 8.16: AP and frog views of pelvis radiographs show congenital hip dislocation in a three-year-old male.

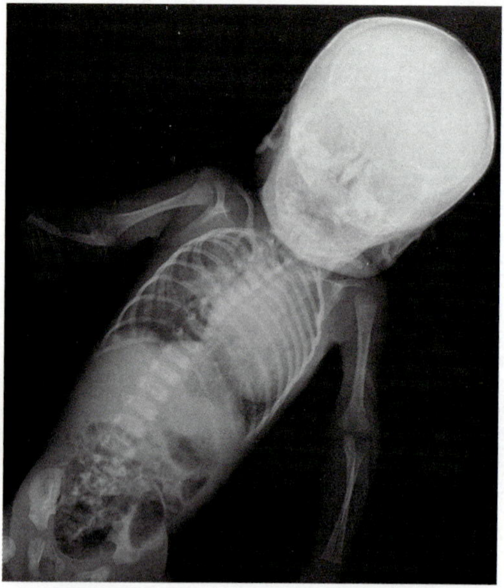

Figure 8.17: Kiddigram shows absent right radius with congenital heart disease—Holt-Oram syndrome.

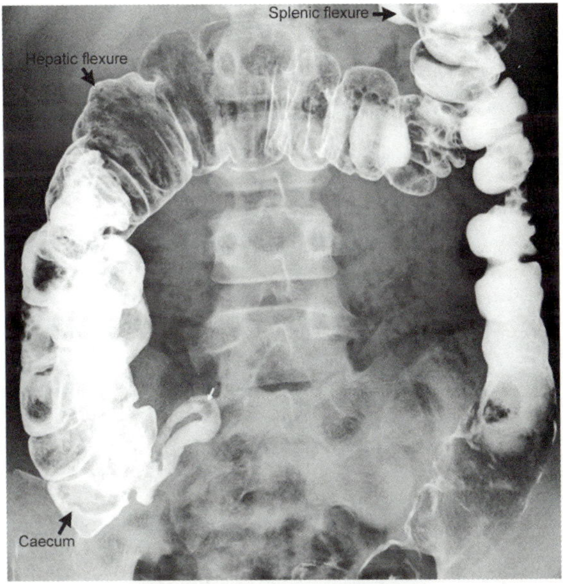

Figure 8.18: Normal appendix (white arrow) and caecum (black arrow) on barium enema examination.

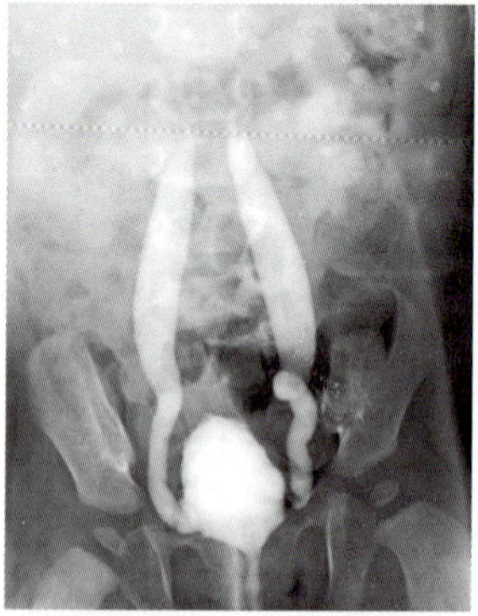

Figure 8.19: Grade 5 vesico-ureteric reflux in an eight-month-old female child.

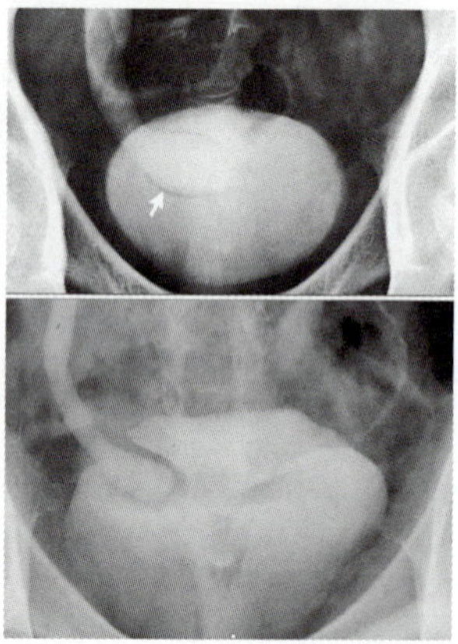

Figure 8.20: Intravenous urogram shows ureterocele (cobra head appearance) on right side (arrow) in two different patients.

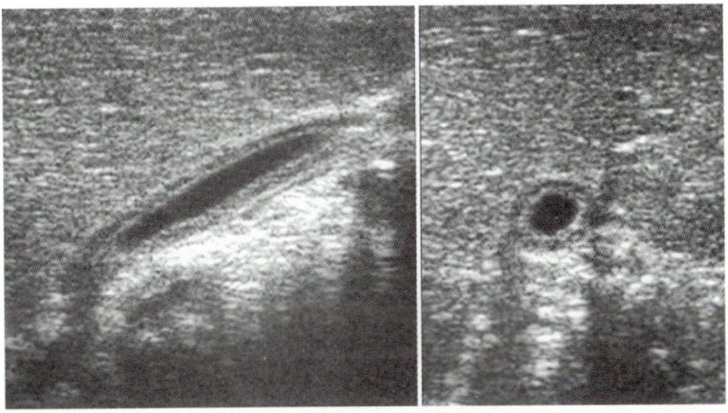

Figure 8.21: Ultrasound appearance of normal post-feed gallbladder in an infant.

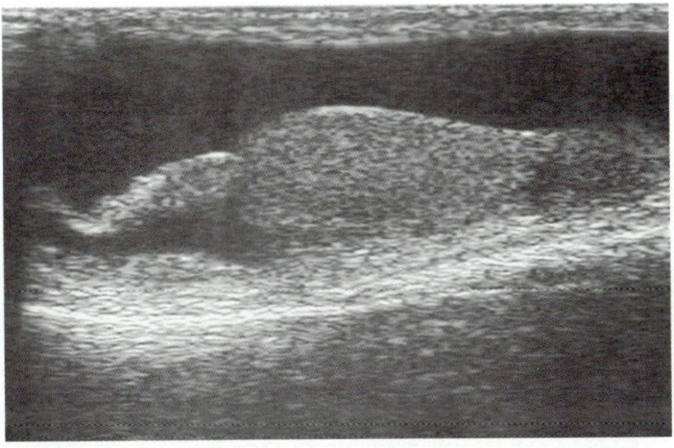

Figure 8.22: Ultrasound shows congenital hydrocele in a six-year-old child.

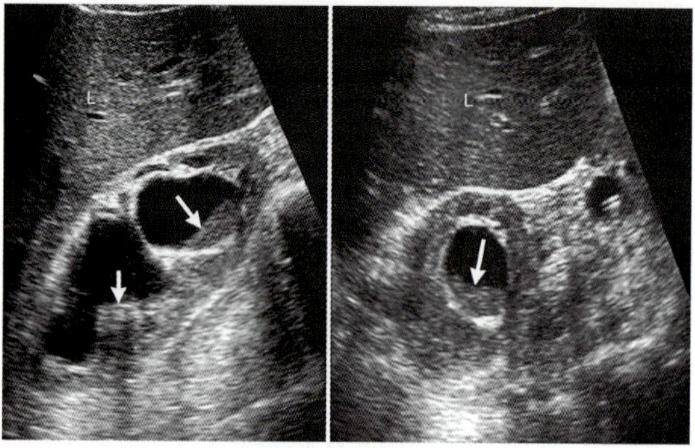

Figure 8.23: Enlarged hydronephrotic kidney with a fluid-fluid levels (arrows) in the dilated calyces secondary to pus appearing as echogenic debris in a case of pyohydronephrosis.

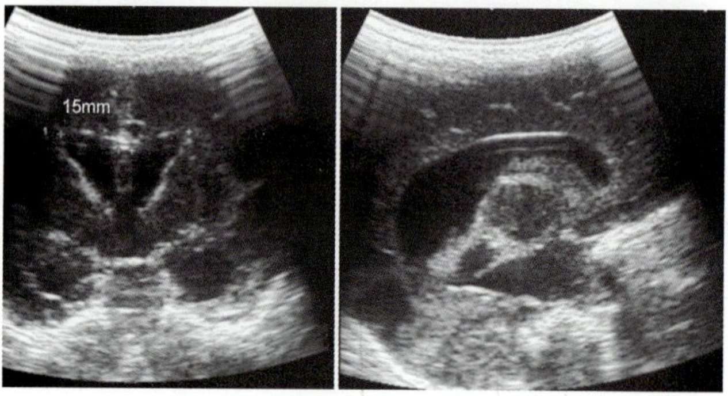

Figure 8.24: Ultrasound images through anterior fontanelle show dilated lateral ventricles in 40-day-old child.

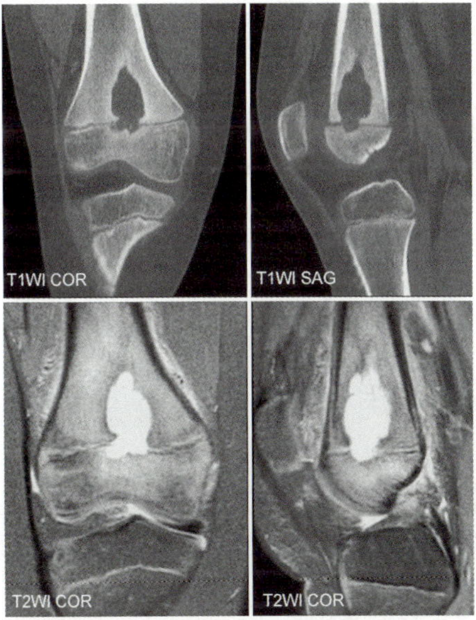

Figure 8.25: Brodie's abscess lower end of femur extending into the epiphysis on MRI.

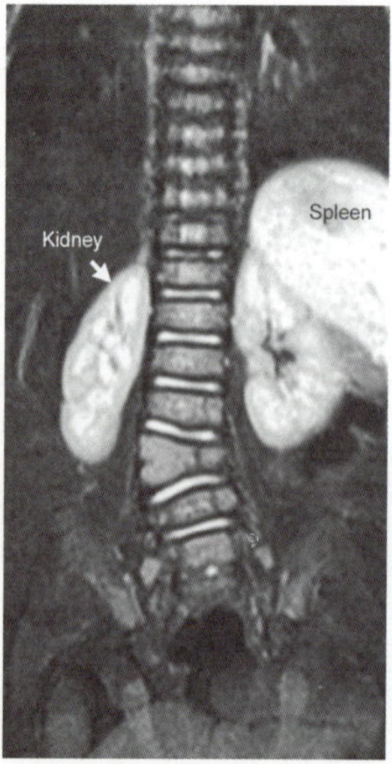

Figure 8.26: Lumbar hemivertebrae in a one-year-old male child on coronal MRI.

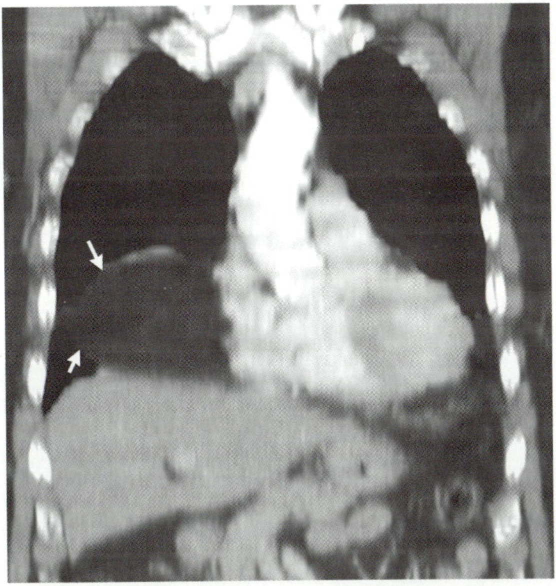

Figure 8.27: Coronal reconstructed CT image shows a large epicardial fat pad (arrow) in right cardiophrenic angle, a normal variant.

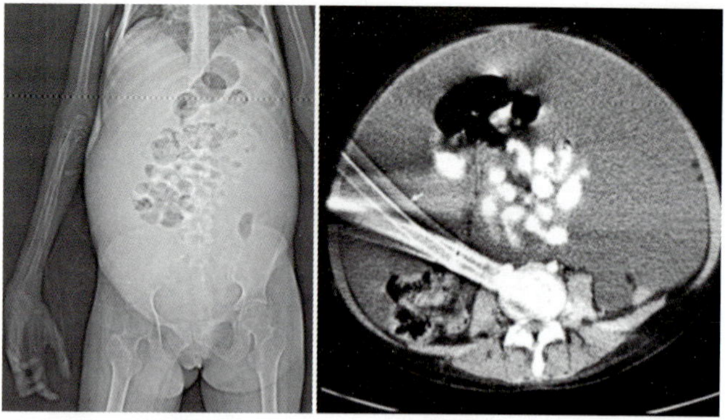

Figure 8.28: Motion artifact due to accidental motion of right forearm (arrow) being brought anterior to abdomen by the child during CT scan. Massive ascites is present.

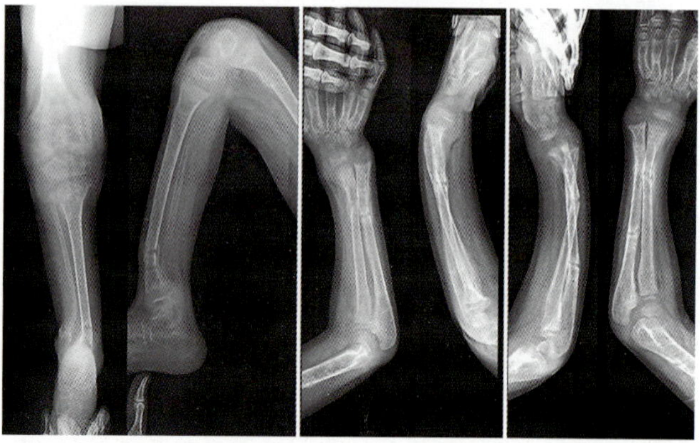

Figure 8.29: X-ray both legs and forearms in a case of osteogenesis imperfecta show pathological fractures.

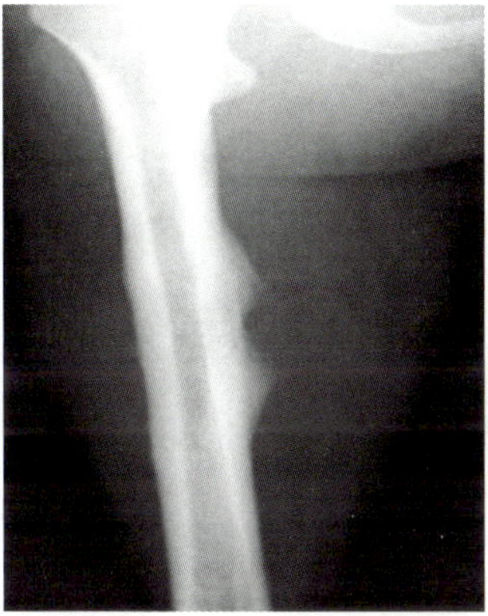

Figure 8.30: X-ray right thigh, the femoral shaft shows periosteal with soft tissue swelling suggesting Ewings sarcoma.

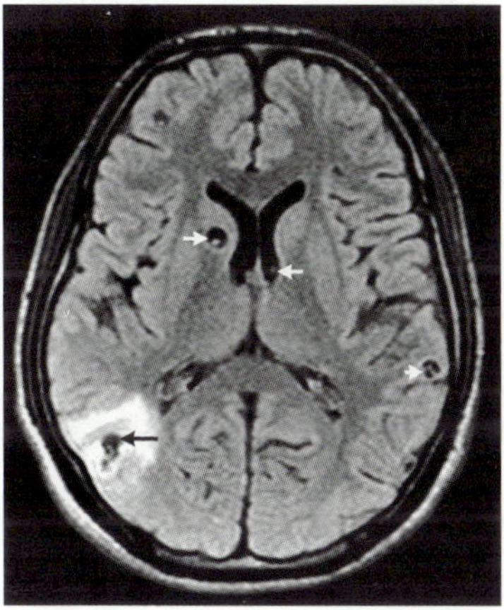

Figure 8.31: MR image shows multiple cysticercosis cysts (arrow) in which the scolex can be appreciated. The long arrow shows cyst with surrounding edema. White arrow shows the scolex of intraventricular cyst.

OSSIFICATION CENTERS

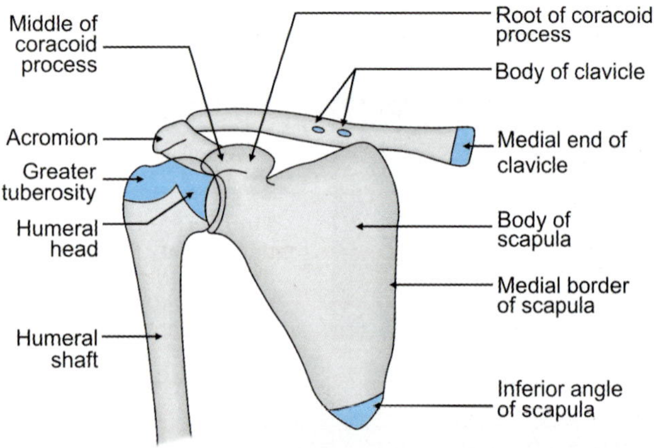

Figure 8.32: Shoulder joint

Shoulder Joint

BONES	OSSIFICATION
Body of Scapula	8th week of fetal life
Body of Clavicle (two centers)	5th and 6th week of fetal life
Shaft of Humerus	8th week of fetal life

EPIPHYSIS	APPEARANCE	FUSION
Head of Humerus	1 year	
Greater Tuberosity	3 years	
Lesser Tuberosity	5 years	
Acromian Process	15–18 years	25th year
Middle of Coracoid Process	1 year	15th year
Root of Coracoid Process	17 years	25th year
Inferior Angle of Scapula	14–20 years	22–25 years
Medial Border of Scapula	14–20 years	22–25 years
Medial End of Clavicle	18–20 years	25th year

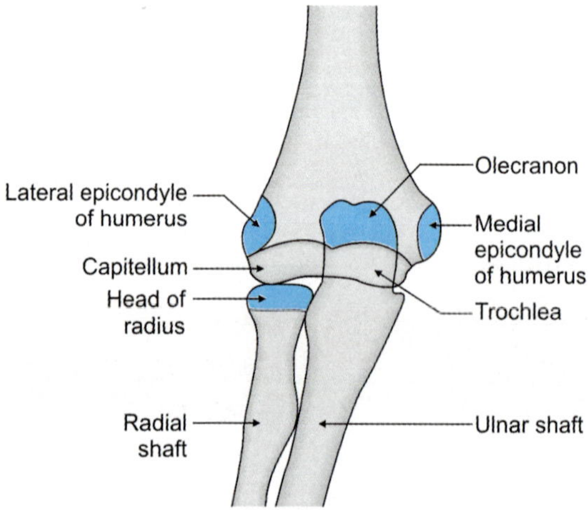

Figure 8.33: Elbow joint

Elbow Joint

BONES	OSSIFICATION
Radial Shaft	8th week of fetal life
Ulnar Shaft	8th week of fetal life

EPIPHYSIS	APPEARANCE	FUSION
Lateral Epicondyle	10–12 years	17–18 years
Medial Epicondyle	05–08 years	17–18 years
Capitellum	01–03 years	17–18 years
Head of Radius	05–06 years	16–19 years
Trochlea	11th year	18th year
Olecranon Process	10–13 years	16–20 years

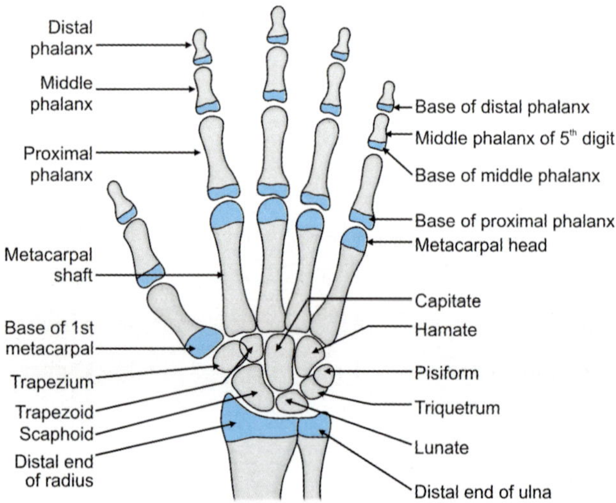

Figure 8.34: Wrist and hand

Wrist and Hand

BONES	OSSIFICATION
Capitate	4 months
Hamate	4 months
Triquetrum	3 years
Lunate	4–5 years
Trapezium	6 years
Trapezoid	6 years
Pisiform	11 years
Metacarpals	10th week of fetal life
Proximal Phalanges	11th week of fetal life
Middle Phalanges	12th week of fetal life
Distal Phalanges	9th week of fetal life
Middle Phalanx of 5th Digit	14th week of fetal life

EPIPHYSIS	APPEARANCE	FUSION
Lower End of Radius	1–2 years	20th year
Lower End of Ulna	5–8 years	20th year
Metacarpal Heads	2.5 years	20th year
Base of Proximal Phalanges	2.5 years	20th year
Base of Middle Phalanges	3 years	18–20 years
Base of Distal Phalanges	3 years	18–20 years
Base of 1st Metacarpal	2.5 years	20th year

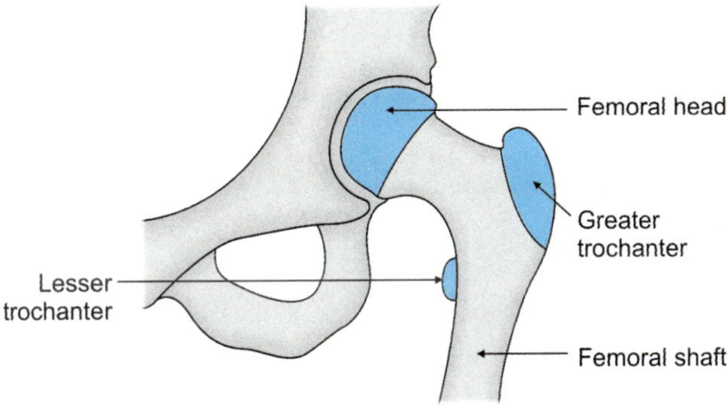

Figure 8.35: Hip joint

Hip Joint

BONES	OSSIFICATION
Proximal Femoral Shaft	7th week of fetal life

EPIPHYSIS	APPEARANCE	FUSION
Femoral Head	1 year	18–20 years
Greater Trochanter	3–5 years	18–20 years
Lesser Trochanter	8–14 years	18–20 years

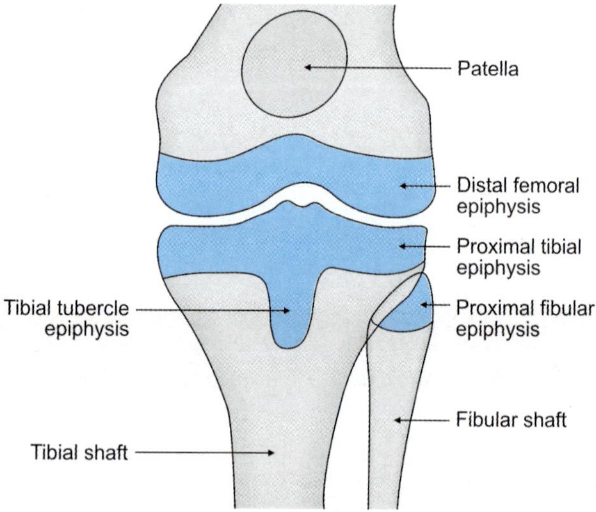

Figure 8.36: Knee joint

Knee Joint

BONES	OSSIFICATION
Tibial Shaft	7th week of fetal life
Fibular Shaft	8th week of fetal life
Patella	5 years

EPIPHYSIS	APPEARANCE	FUSION
Proximal Tibia	At birth	20th year
Tibial Tubercle	5–10 years	20th year
Proximal Fibular	4th year	25th year
Distal Femoral	At birth	20th year

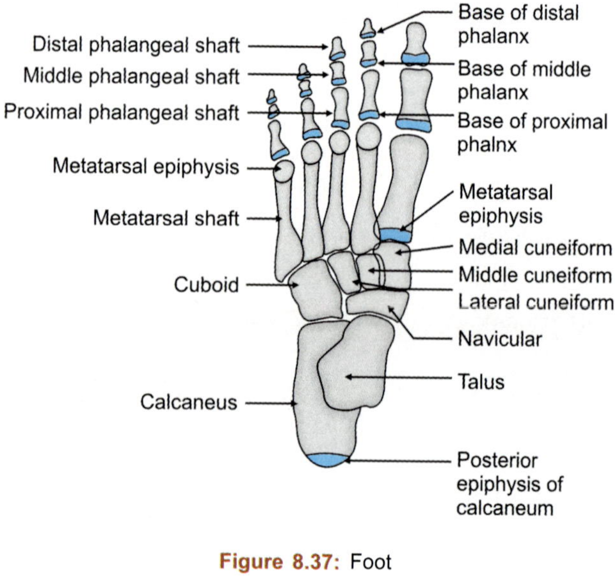

Figure 8.37: Foot

Foot

BONES	OSSIFICATION
Calcaneus	6th month of fetal life
Talus	6th month of fetal life
Navicular	3–4 years
Cuboid	At birth
Lateral Cuneiform	1 year
Middle Cuneiform	3 years
Medial Cuneiform	3 years
Metatarsal Shafts	8th–9th week of fetal life
Phalangeal Shafts	10th week of fetal life

EPIPHYSIS	APPEARANCE	FUSION
Metatarsals	3 years	17–20 years
Proximal Phalangeal Base	3 years	17–20 years
Middle Phalangeal Base	3 years	17–20 years
Distal Phalangeal Base	5 years	17–20 years
Posterior Calcaneal	5 years	At puberty

PHYSICAL PRINCIPLE OF CT SCAN IMAGING

CT was invented in 1972 by British engineer, Sir Godfrey Newbold Hounsfield in Hayes, United Kingdom at EMI Central Research Laboratories using X-rays. EMI Laboratories is best known today for its music and recording business. About the same time South Africa-born American physicist, Allan McLeod Cormack of Tufts University in Massachusetts independently invented a similar process, and both shared the 1979 Nobel Prize.

The first clinical CT scan was installed in 1974. The initial systems were dedicated only to head scanning due to small gantry, but soon this was overcome and whole body CT system with larger gantry became available in 1976.

Basic principle is to obtain a tomogram having thickness in millimeters of the region of interest using pencil beam X-radiation. The radiation transmitted through the patient is counted by scintillation detector. This information when fed in the computer is analyzed by mathematical algorithms and reconstructed as a tomographic image by the computer so as to provide an insight into the structure being studied.

DEVELOPMENTS IN CT TECHNOLOGY

Conventional Axial CT

Table 8.1: Generations of CT scan

Generation of CT scan	*Motion of X-ray tube-detector system*	*Stationary detectors*	*X-ray beam type*
First	Translate-Rotate	Two detectors	Pencil beam
Second	Translate-Rotate	Multiple detectors upto 30	Narrow fan beam (10°)
Third	Rotate-Rotate	Multiple detectors upto 750	Wide fan beam (50°)
Fourth	Rotate-Fixed	Ring of 1500–4500 detectors	Fan beam

Spiral/Helical CT

Spiral CT uses the conventional technology in conjunction with slip ring technology, which simultaneously provides high voltage for X-ray tube, low voltage for control unit and transmits digital data from detector array. Slip ring is a circular instrument with sliding bushes that enables the gantry to rotate continuously while the patient table moves into the gantry simultaneously, thus three-dimensional volume rendered image can be obtained. The advantages over the conventional scanner are the reduced scan time, reduced radiation exposure and reduced contrast requirement with superior information.

Electron Beam CT (EBCT)

In EBCT, both the X-ray source and the detectors are stationary. High energy focused electron beam is magnetically steered on the tungsten target to emit X-rays which pass through the subject on to the detectors and image is acquired. EBCT is particularly used for faster imaging in cardiac studies.

Multislice/Multidetector CT (MDCT)

Spiral CT uses single row of detectors, resulting in a single slice per gantry rotation. Multislice CT, multiple detector arrays are used resulting in multiple slices per gantry rotation. In addition, fan beam geometry of spiral CT is replaced by cone beam geometry.

The major advantages over spiral CT are improved spatial and temporal resolution, reduced image noise, faster and longer anatomic coverage and increased concentration of intravenous contrast.

Dual Source CT

The dual energy technology of the new Flash CT provides higher contrast between normal and abnormal tissues making it easier to see abnormalities while reducing radiation. With its two rotating X-ray tubes, enhanced speed and power allows children to be screened more effectively. It turns off the radiation when it comes close to sensitive tissue areas of the body like thyroid, breasts, or eye lens.

Pediatric patients benefit because they do not need to hold breath or lay completely still during the examination and they do not have to be sedated.

Hounsfield Units

CT numbers recognized by the computer are from (–) 1000 to (+) 1000, i.e. a range of 2000 Hounsfield units which are present in the image as 2000 shades of gray, but our eye cannot precisely discriminate between these 2000 different shades.

Hounsfield scale assigns attenuation value of water as zero (HU 0). And other tissues their attenuation value as compared to water is:

Table 8.2: Attenuation value of various tissues on CT scan

Tissue	Attenuation value in HU
Air	(–)1000
Lung	(–) 400 to (–) 800
Fat	(–) 40 to (–) 100
Water	0
Fresh blood	55 to 65
Soft tissue	40 to 80
Bone	400 to 1000

Window Level (WL) and Window Width (WW)

To permit the viewer to understand the image, only a restricted number of HU are put on view and this is accomplished by setting the WL and WW on the console to a suitable range of Hounsfield units, depending on the tissue, for interpreting the image. The expression WL represents the central Hounsfield value of all the Hounsfield numbers within the WW. Tissues with CT numbers outside this array are shown as either black of white. Both the WL and WW can be set on the displayed image as desired by the viewer. On CT examination of the chest, a WW of 300 to 350 and WL of 35 to 45 are chosen to image the mediastinum (soft tissue window) whereas WW of 1500 and WL of 0 is used to assess the lung window.

Image Reconstruction

The acquisition of volumetric data using spiral CT means that the images can be postprocessed in ways appropriate to the clinical situation.

Multiplanar reformatting (MPR) is taking by standard axial images and subject to the three-dimensional array of CT numbers obtained with a series of contiguous slices; and can be viewed in sagittal, coronal, oblique and paraxial planes (Figures 8.38A to C).

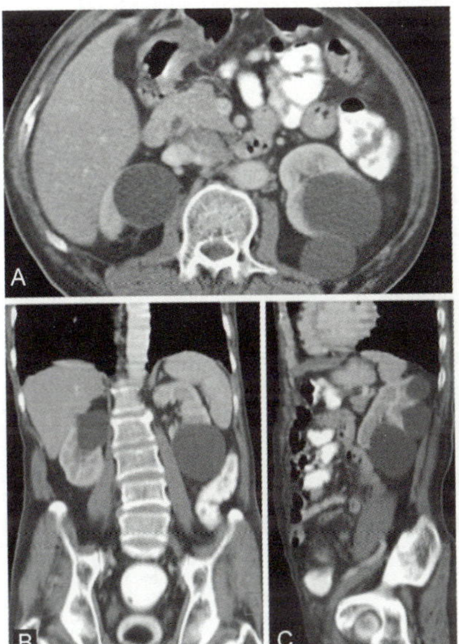

Figures 8.38A to C: Bilateral renal cysts seen in axial section (A) are reformatted into sagittal (B) and coronal (C) planes.

Three-Dimensional Imaging

Many fractures like facial fractures can be reconstructed into a 3-dimensional image (Figures 8.39A to D) for superior surgical evaluationand understanding.

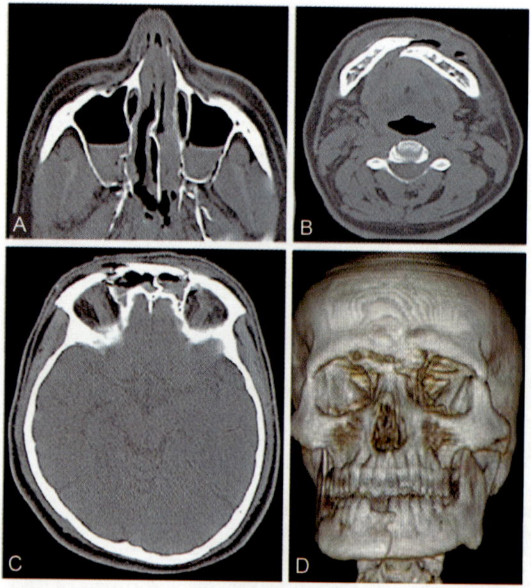

Figures 8.39A to D: Fracture of body of mandible and frontal bone. With bilateral maxillary hemosinus. D shows the 3D image of face including mandible.

CT Angiography

CT angiography (CTA) technique is created subsequent to intravenous contrast, images are acquired in the arterial phase and then reconstructed and exhibited in 2D or 3D format. This performance is used for imaging the aorta, renal, cerebral, coronary and peripheral arteries (Figures 8.40A to D and 8.41, 8.42).

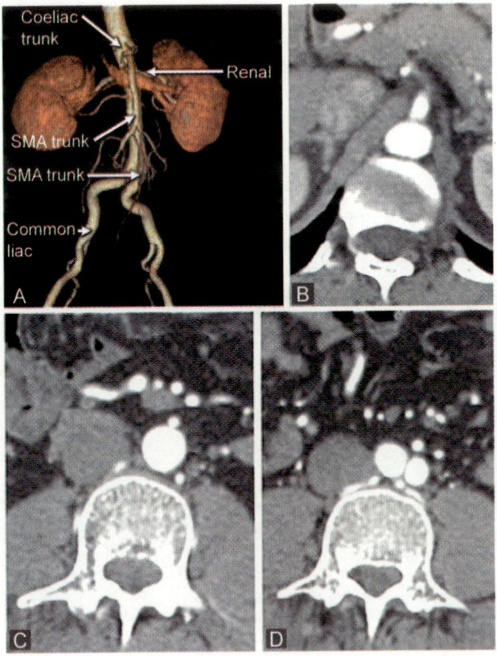

Figures 8.40A to D: CT abdominal angiography (anterior).

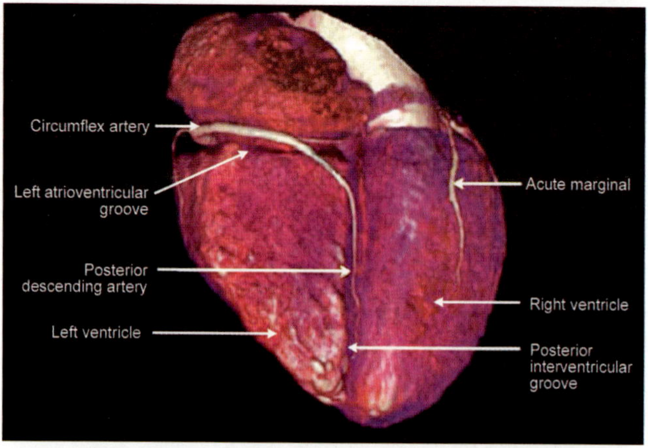

Figure 8.41: Volume rendered image posterior coronal plane shows coronary arteries.

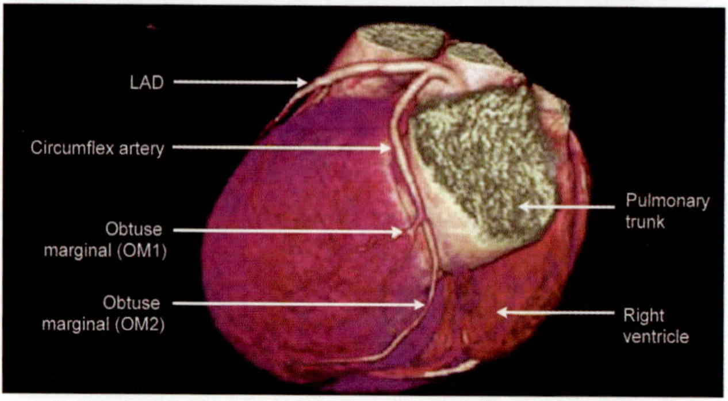

Figure 8.42: Volume rendered image posterior oblique coronal plane shows coronary arteries

CT is readily available in most hospitals and stand-alone CT centers. It is fast imaging modality and provides with cross sectional high resolution images. Data acquired on axial scans can be used for multiplanar and 3D reconstructions. It detects subtle differences between body tissues. However it uses X-rays which have radiation hazards, CT need contrast media for enhanced soft tissue contrast. Contrast is contraindicated in asthma, cardiac disease, renal and certain thyroid conditions.

CT CONTRAST MEDIA

Iodinated Intravascular Agents

Intravascular radiological contrast media are iodine containing chemicals which add to the details from any given CT scan study and thereby aid the diagnosis. They were first introduced by Moses Swick. Iodine (atomic weight 127) is an ideal choice element for X-ray absorption because the korn (K) shell binding energy of iodine (33.7) is nearest to the mean energy used in diagnostic radiography and thus maximum photoelectric interactions can be obtained which are a must for best image quality. These compounds after intravascular injection are rapidly distributed by capillary permeability into extravascular-extracellular space and almost 90% is excreted via glomerular filtration by kidneys within 12 hours.

Following iodinated contrast media are available:

1. Ionic monomers, e.g. diatrizoate, iothamalate, metrizoate.
2. Nonionic monomers, e.g. iohexol, iopamidol, iomeron.
3. Ionic dimer, e.g. ioxaglate.
4. Nonionic dimer, e.g. Iodixanol, Iotrolan.

The amount of contrast required is usually 1–2 ml/kg body weight. Normal osmolality of human serum is 290 mOsm/kg. Ionic contrast media have much higher osmolality than normal human serum and are known as High Osmolar Contrast Media (HOCM), while nonionic contrast media have lower osmolality than normal human serum and are known as Low Osmolar Contrast Media (LOCM).

Side effects or adverse reactions to contrast media are divided as:

1. Idiosyncratic anaphylactoid reactions.
2. Nonidiosyncratic reactions like nephrotoxicity and cardiotoxicity.

Adverse reactions are more with HOCM than LOCM. So LOCM are preferred. Delayed adverse reactions although very rare but more common with LOCM and include iodide mumps, systemic lupus erythematosus (SLE) and Stevens-Johnson syndrome. Principles of treatment of adverse reaction involves mainly five basic steps: ABCDE

A – Maintain proper airway.

B – Breathing—Support for adequate breathing.

C – Maintain adequate circulation. Obtain an IV access.

D – Use of appropriate drugs like antihistaminics for urticaria, atropine for vasovagal hypotension and bradycardia, beta agonists for bronchospasm, hydrocortisone, etc.

E – Always have emergency back-up ready including ICU care.

Following intravascular iodinated agent arterial opacification takes place at approximately 20 seconds with venous peak at approximately 70 seconds. The level then declines and the contrast is finally excreted by the kidneys. These different phases of enhancement are used to image various organs depending on the indication. Spiral CT, being faster is able to acquire images during each phase, thus providing much more information.

ORAL CONTRAST

The bowel is usually opacified in CT examinations of the abdomen and pelvis as the attenuation value of the bowel is similar to the surrounding structures and as a result pathological lesions can be obscured. Materials used include barium or iodine based preparations, which are given to the patient to drink preceding the examination to opacify the gastrointestinal tract.

Barium Sulphate

Barium sulphate preparations are used for evaluating gastrointestinal tract. Barium (atomic weight 137) is an ideal choice element for X-ray absorption because the K shell binding energy of barium (37) is near to the mean energy used in diagnostic radiography and thus maximum photoelectric interactions can be obtained which are a must for best image quality. Moreover, barium sulphate is nonabsorbable, nontoxic and can be prepared into a stable suspension. For CT scan of abdomen, 1000–1500 mL of 1–5% w/vol barium sulphate suspension can be used. Adverse reactions are rare. Rarely, mediastinal leakage can lead to fibrosing mediastinitis while peritoneal leakage can cause adhesive peritonitis.

Iodinated Agents

Iodine containing oral contrast agents like Gastrografin and Trazograf are given for evaluating gastrointestinal tract on CT scan.

Air

Air is used as a negative per rectal contrast medium in large bowel during CT abdomen and during CT colonography.

Carbon Dioxide

Rarely carbon dioxide is used for infradiaphragmatic CT angiography in patients who are sensitive to iodinated contrast.

PHYSICAL PRINCIPLE OF MAGNETIC RESONANCE IMAGING

Magnetic resonance imaging (MRI) is based on the principle of electromagnetic character of atomic nuclei which was first described by physicist Felix Bloch and Edward Purcell in 1946. They received a Noble prize for this in 1952. However it was long after this that nuclear magnetic resonance was used for imaging. In 1973, Lauterbur showed that images of human body could be acquired by placing a magnetic field around it. First human images were published by Damadian et al in 1977. Since then use of MRI for medical imaging has seen an exponential growth and now it is a mainstay in the field of medical diagnostics.

Electromagnetism is at the core of MRI physics. When current is passed through a wire, a magnetic field is created around it. Similarly, in a nucleus with odd number of protons or neutrons, the electrons rotating around the nucleus produce a field around them. This gives a "charge" to the nucleus, also called as the spinning charge or "the spin". Thus these nuclei behave as tiny magnets. Hydrogen proton is the most favorable nucleus for MRI as it is widely available in the water molecules present in the body.

When these nuclei are placed in an external magnetic field (B_0), they either align along the magnetic field or against it. When the number of nuclei along the magnetic field is more as compared to those against the field, a net magnetization is created in the direction of the field.

In order to generate a signal from these spinning nuclei, they have to be tipped out of alignment with B_0 (i.e. out of the longitudinal plane and towards the transverse plane). The signal generated by each rotating nucleus is much stronger if the nuclei precess in unison with each other at 90 degrees to the main magnetic field. For this, a second magnetic field is introduced and it is referred to as B_1. This B_1 should be applied perpendicular to B_0, and it has to be at the resonant frequency. Radiofrequency (RF) coils are used to transmit B_1. If sufficient RF pulse is applied, the spins are flipped into the transverse plane. This is the 90° RF pulse and it generates the strongest signal. However as this is a high energy state, the signal starts decaying quickly and is called free induction decay (FID). This decay or relaxation is of two types:

T1 relaxation—It is the relaxation in the longitudinal plane due to the spins returning to the normal equilibrium state and aligning with the main magnetic field.

T2 relaxation—There is dephasing in the transverse plane (90 degree plane). Each individual proton precesses at slightly different speed. After a while, the signal from protons in transverse plane degenerates as protons start precessing out of phase with each other. This is T2 relaxation.

In human tissue, T1 is usually 10 times longer than T2 which means that T2 decay occurs before T1 recovery. In actual practice, the T2 dephasing time is much quicker than the 'natural' T2 due to inhomogeneities in the magnetic field B_0. This reduced T2 is called T2*.

T1W and T2W images result by manipulating the manner and frequency in which RF pulses are applied

(Time to Repetition–TR), and by changing time to start of signal acquisition after RF has been applied (Time to Echo—TE), T1-weighted or T2-weighted images can be obtained.

Pulse sequences: (1) Partial saturation (PS): It is also known as gradient echo or field echo and it uses a 90° RF pulse. (2) Spin echo (SE): A 90° pulse is followed by 180° refocusing RF pulse. (3) Inversion recovery (IR): 180° pulse is followed by a 90° pulse.

In a typical image acquisition, the basic unit of each sequence (i.e. the 90°–180°—signal detection) is repeated hundreds of times. By altering the time to echo (TE) or time to repetition (TR), i.e. the time between successive 90° pulses, the signal contrast can be altered or weighted. For example, if a long TE is used, inherent differences in T2 times of tissues will become apparent. Tissues with a long T2 (e.g. water) will take longer to decay and their signal will be greater (or appear brighter in the image) than the signal from tissue with a short T2 (e.g. fat). In a similar manner TR governs T1 contrast. Tissue with a long TR (water) will take a long time to recover back to the equilibrium magnetization value, therefore a short TR interval will make this tissue appear dark compared to tissue with a short T1 (fat). When TE and TR are chosen to minimize both these weightings, the signal contrast is only derived from the number or density of spins in a given tissue. This image is said to be proton density weighted (PDW).

Table 8.3: Time to Echo and Time to Repetition for MR sequences

	Echo Time TE	*Repetition Time TR*
T1 Weighted or T1W	Long TE	Long TR
T2-Weighted or T2W	Short TE	Short TR
Proton Density Weighted or PDW	Short TE	Long TR

Table 8.4: Signal intensity of various tissues at T1, T2 and Proton Density imaging

Tissue	*T1*	*T2*	*Proton Density*
Fat	Bright	Bright (less than T1)	Bright
Water	Dark	Bright	Intermediate bright
Cerebral Gray Matter	Gray	Gray	Gray
Cerebral White Matter	White	Dark	Dark
TR Values TE Values	TR > 1500 TE < 50	TR > 1500 TE > 80	TR > 1500 TE < 50

Air is black in all sequences because of very few protons and cortical bone is always black due to no mobility of protons.

Each volume element in the body has a different resonant frequency which depends on the protons present within it. This produces a signal which is specific to the resonant frequency of that volume element. This signal is analyzed by the computer using a mathematical technique called as Fourier analysis.

Magnet forms the main component of the MRI, it is of two types: (1) Permanent or resistive magnets used in low field scanners and are usually referred to as open MRI. (2) Superconducting magnet used in scanners above 1.0 Tesla. It is made from an alloy usually Niobium and Titanium (Nb-Ti) that has zero electrical resistance below a critical temperature. To maintain this temperature the magnet is enclosed and cooled by a cryogen containing liquid helium which has to be topped-up on a regular basis.

RF coils are needed to transmit and/or receive the MR signal. The RF coil should cover only the volume of interest. This gives an optimal signal-to-noise ratio (SNR). To achieve this there are various types of RF coils with trade-offs in terms of coverage and sensitivity, e.g. head coil being smaller in size provides better SNR. Body coil is integrated into the scanner bore and is not seen by the patient. Both these coils act as transceivers, i.e. they transmit and receive. Surface coils are used for imaging anatomy near to the coil. They are simple loop designs and have excellent SNR when close to the coil but the sensitivity drops off rapidly with distance from the coil. These are only used as receivers, the body coil acting as the transmitter. Quadrature or circularly-polarized coils comprise of two coils 90° apart to improve SNR by a factor of 2½.

Advanced applications include diffusion imaging, perfusion imaging, functional MRI, spectroscopy and interventional MRI.

Possible adverse effects of MRI can be due to static magnetic field, gradients, RF heating, noise and claustrophobia.

Caution needs to be exercised while selecting patients for MRI. Patients with pacemakers, metallic implants, aneurysm clips should not be subjected to MRI. The newer implants are made of MR compatible material like titanium. Metallic objects should not be taken near the magnet as they can be injurious to the patient, personnel and equipment.

Special Sequences

A. Short Tau Inversion Recovery (STIR) Sequence

It is heavily T2 weighted imaging, as a result the fluid and edema return high signal intensity and it annuls out the signal from fluid. The resultant images show the areas of pathology clearly. The sequence is useful in musculoskeletal imaging as it annuls the signal from normal bone marrow.

B. Fluid Attenuated Inversion Recovery (FLAIR)

This is an inversion-recovery pulse sequence that suppresses or annuls out the signal from water. The sequence is useful to show subtle lesions in the brain and spinal cord as it annuls the signal from CSF. It is useful to bring out the periventricular hyperintense lesions, e.g., in multiple sclerosis.

C. Gradient Echo Sequence

This sequence reduces the scan times. This is achieved by giving a shorter RF pulse leading to a lesser amount of disruption to the magnetic vectors. The sequence is useful in identifying calcification and blood degradation products.

D. Diffusion-Weighted Imaging

'Diffusion' portrays the movement of molecules due to random motion. It enables to distinguish between rapid diffusion of protons (unrestricted diffusion) and slow diffusion of protons (restricted diffusion). GRE pulse sequence has been devised to image the diffusion of water through tissues. It is a sensitive way of detecting acute brain infarcts, where diffusion is reduced or restricted.

E. MR Angiography

The most common MR angiographic techniques are time-of-flight imaging and phase contrast. In these sequences, multiple RF pulses are applied with short TRs saturate the spins in stationary tissues. This results in suppression of the signal from stationary tissues in the imaging slab. In-flowing blood is unaffected by the repetitive RF pulses, as a result, as it enters the imaging slab, its signal is not suppressed and appears hyperintense compared with that of stationary tissue. Time-of-flight imaging may be 2D, with section-by-section acquisition, or 3D, with acquisition of a larger volume. MRA can also be performed with intravenous gadolinium when in the vascular phase of enhancement.

MRI CONTRAST

A. Intravenous Contrast Agents

In MRI the most commonly used intravenous contrast agents are gadolinium chelates, the paramagnetic property of gadolinium provides contrast. It has the ability to alter the magnetic characteristics of neighboring tissues. The effect of this is shortening of the T1 and T2 relaxation times. Shortening of T1 effects are exploited since shortening of T1 relaxation time leads to an increase in signal intensity.

Gadolinium containing contrast agents available are *gadodiamide* (Omniscan), *gadobenic acid* (Multihance), *gadopentetic acid* (Magnevist), *gadoteridol* (Prohance), *gadofosveset* (Ablavar), *gadoversetamide* (OptiMARK), *gadoxetic acid* (Eovist or Primovist).

Other MRI contrast agents gaining recognition are superparamagnetic agents, i.e. iron oxide and manganese.

Two types of iron oxide contrast agents exist: *Superparamagnetic* Iron Oxide (SPIO) and Ultrasmall Superparamagnetic Iron Oxide (USPIO). These contrast agents consist of suspended *colloids* of iron oxide *nanoparticles* and are injectables, they reduce the T2 signals of absorbing tissues. SPIO and USPIO contrast agents have been used successfully in some liver tumor enhancement. Available iron oxide contrast agents are Cliavist, Combidex, Resovist and Sinerem.

Manganese chelates such as Mn-DPDP enhance the T1 signal and have been used for the detection of liver lesions. These are absorbed intra-cellularly and excreted in *bile*.

B. Oral Contrast Agents

In MRI oral contrast can be used for enhancement of the gastrointestinal tract. Gadolinium, manganese chelates and iron salts are used for T1 signal enhancement.

SPIO, *barium sulfate*, air and clay have been used to lower T2 signal. *Blueberry* and *green tea* having high manganese concentration can also be used for T1 increasing contrast enhancement.

Perflubron, a type of perfluorocarbon, has been used as a gastrointestinal MRI contrast agent for pediatric imaging. This contrast agent works by reducing the amount of protons in a body cavity.

Gadolinium initially disperses through the vascular system and then diffuses into the extracellular space, before moving into the intracellular space. Whilst still circulating within the vessels, magnetic resonance angiography (MRA) can be performed.

Gadolinium does not cross the intact blood-brain barrier but helps identifying intracranial lesions with interruption of the barrier, like infection and tumors. It helps to discriminate tumors from edema, low-grade from high-grade tumors, scar tissue from tumor tissue.

Oral gadolinium is used to highlight loops of bowel to distinguish from surrounding soft tissue.

Superparamagnetic agents are more specific for hepatic lesions and are specially taken up by the Kupffer cells in the liver and help make a distinction between normal liver and malignant tissue.

MRA

All pulse sequences are sensitive to flow. There is a complex relationship between the type and rate of flow and the resultant signal intensity. As a general rule, fast or turbulent vascular flow results in a signal dropout, whilst slow vascular flow results in high signal. There are two principal flow-sensitive sequences, time of flight and phase contrast. MRA can also be performed with intravenous gadolinium whilst in the vascular phase of enhancement.

Ultrasonography (USG)

Diagnostic ultrasound is a noninvasive imaging modality utilizing high frequency sound energy in the range of 3 to 15 megahertz (MHz). This is well above the normal human ear response to sound frequency of 20–20,000 Hz.

USG works on piezoelectric effect of crystals made from lead zirconate titanate or polyvinylidene difluoride and is used in forming images by using pulse echo principle. Gray scale (B) mode is used in general imaging. Motion (M) mode is used for echocardiography. Color Doppler ultrasound is used for imaging of vessels; Christian Doppler was first to put forth the principle of Doppler.

High frequency sound waves travel through human tissue; they are reflected on traversing interfaces. A transducer which emits high frequency sound is moved over the patient; the reflected waves are returned to the transducer resulting in an image by the computer.

Echoes or reflections of the ultrasound beam form interfaces between tissues with different acoustic properties, resulting in information on the size, shape and structure of organ or mass. Ultrasound is largely reflected by air-soft tissue interface and bone-soft tissue interface, thus being of relatively limited use in the chest and musculoskeletal system.

Ultrasonography does not use X-rays, as a result there is no risk of ionizing radiations. It is real time, permits multiplanar imaging, helps positive decision for a lesion to be cystic or solid. It is used to perform interventional procedures. The equipment is portable, inexpensive, easily available and low risk. It is low cost, being cheaper than other cross-sectional imaging techniques. *Doppler evaluation allows analysis of blood flow*. There are no known harmful effects of *high frequency sound waves* on human body.

Disadvantages of USG are few. It is difficult in obese patients and in viewing deep structures; it does not show function of tissues. Air, bone and fat are enemies to good ultrasound imaging.

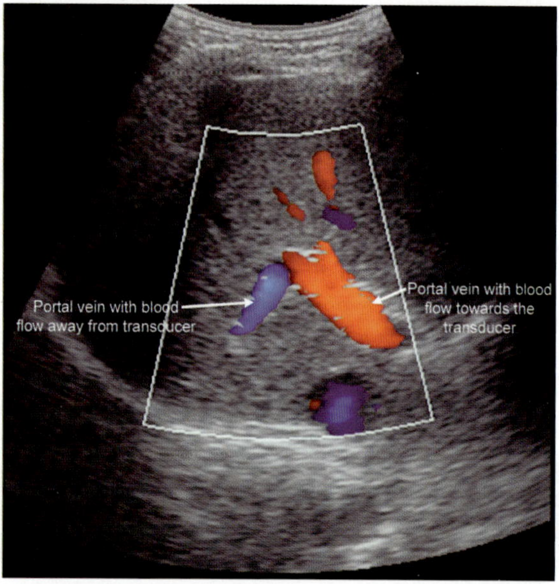

Figure 8.43: Liver image, a Doppler interrogation box placed over the portal vein.

Doppler ultrasonography employs the frequency shift in the reflected ultrasonic beam to recognize the moving fluid in the body. It demonstrates the presence and direction of blood flow. It gives red color coding for blood flowing towards the transducer and blue coding to blood flowing away from the transducer (Figure 8.43). Doppler can be used to attain spectral trace that shows velocity of flow.

Ultrasound Contrast

Ultrasound contrast agents comprise of gas-filled *microbubbles* measuring less than five microns are given intravenously. Microbubbles have a high degree of echogenicity and ability to reflect the ultrasound waves. The echogenicity difference between the gas in the microbubbles and the soft *tissue* surroundings is immense. Thereby, microbubble contrast agents enhance the ultrasound reflections to produce a high echogenicity difference image. Contrast-enhanced ultrasound can be used to image blood *perfusion* in organs and measure *blood flow* rate in the *heart* and other organs.

Optison or Levovist, are injected intravenously into the systemic circulation in a small bolus. The microbubbles remain in the systemic circulation for a certain period of time. During that time, ultrasound waves are directed on the area of interest. The microbubbles reflect unique *echo* that stands out in contrast to the surrounding tissue. The ultrasound system converts the strong echogenicity into a contrast-enhanced image of the area of interest. Similarly the bloodstream's echo is enhanced, thus allowing to distinguish *blood* from surrounding tissues.

Ultrasound imaging allows real-time evaluation of blood flow. Since microbubbles can generate such strong signals, a lower intravenous dosage is needed in micrograms. However microbubbles don't last very long in circulation. They have low circulation time.

The gas inside the shell may be either air or gas (perfluorocarbons), which are liquid at room temperature but gas at body temperature. The large molecules of perfluorocarbons have slow diffusion and solubility which increase the enhancement time of the contrast medium as compared to air. They are less than 5 microns in size. This is important because they must filter out through the smallest capillary, particularly small enough to pass through the pulmonary circulation and the cardiac chambers without disruption. They are stable enough to persist during the examination. The gas or air (almost 100%) is eliminated from the body through the lungs during normal breathing in 15 minutes. This contrast moves about only in the blood confined to vascular space and does not enter the tissues. These microbubbles enhance the blood in a given vessel and demonstrate the pathology. The components of the shell are absorbed by the blood and later metabolized by the liver. There are no proven side effects; they are safe and non-toxic.

PICTURE ARCHIVING AND COMMUNICATION SYSTEM (PACS)

Picture archival and communication system (PACS), is based on universal DICOM (Digital Imaging and Communications in Medicine) format. DICOM solutions are capable of storing and retrieving multi-modality images in a proficient and secure manner, and in assisting and improving hospital workflow and patient diagnosis.

PACS help eliminating paper requisition forms and radiology reports with smooth integration of PACS with existing image acquisition systems.

The aim of PACS is to replace conventional radiographs and reports with a completely electronic network, these digital images can be viewed on monitors in the radiology department, emergency rooms, inpatient and outpatient departments, thus saving time, improving efficiency of hospital and avoiding of incurring the cost of hard copy images in a busy hospital. The three basic means of rendering plain radiographs images to digital are computed radiography (CR) using photostimulable phosphor plate technology; direct digital radiography (DDR) and digitizing conventional analog films. Non-image data, such as scanned documents like PDF (portable document format) is also incorporated in DICOM format. Dictation of reports can be integrated into the system. The recording is automatically sent to a transcript writer's workstation for typing and can also be made available for access by physicians, avoiding typing delays for urgent results.

Among all clinical specialties, radiology has led the way in developing PACS to its present high standards. PACS consists of four major components: the imaging modalities such as radiography, computed radiography, endoscopy, mammography, ultrasound , CT, MRI, PET-CT and MR PET a secured network for the transmission of patient information; workstations for interpreting and reviewing images and archives for the storage and retrieval of images and reports. Backup copy of patient images is provisioned in case images are lost from the PACS. There are several methods for backup storage of images, but they typically involve automatically sending copies of the images to a separate computer for storage, preferably off-site.

In PACS, no patient is irradiated simply because a previous radiograph or CT scan has been lost; the image once acquired onto the PACS is always available when needed. Simultaneous multilocation viewing of the same image is possible on any workstation connected to the PACS. Numerous post processing soft copy manipulations are possible on the viewing monitor. Film packets are no longer an issue with PACS as it provides a filmless solution for all images. PACS can be integrated into the local area network and images from remote villages are sent to the tertiary hospital for reporting (Figure 8.44).

PACS is an expensive investment initially but the costs can be recovered over a 5-year period. It requires dedicated maintenance. It is important to train the doctors, technicians, nurses and other staff to use PACS effectively. Once PACS is fully operational, no films are issued to patients.

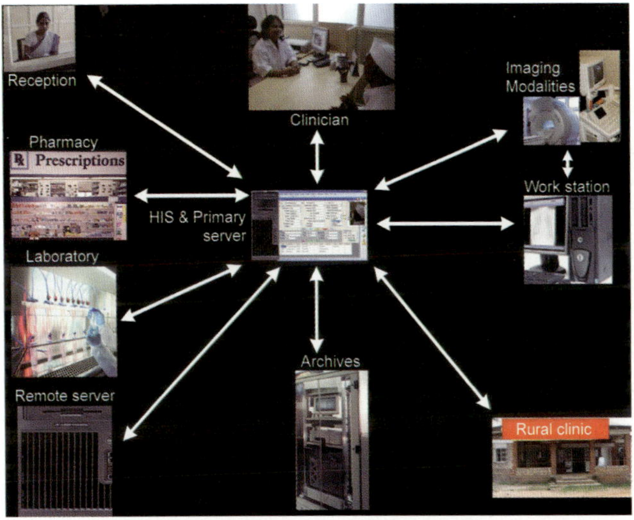

Figure 8.44: PACS flow chart.

PACS breaks the physical and time barriers associated with traditional film-based image retrieval, distribution, and display. PACS can be linked to the internet, leading to teleradiology, the advantages of which are that images can be reviewed from home when on call, can provide linkage between two or more hospitals, outsourcing of imaging examinations in understaffed hospitals. PACS is offered by virtually all the major medical imaging equipment manufacturers, medical IT companies and many independent software companies.

RADIATION SAFETY MEASURES

Radiation is a form of energy which can travel from one place to another even in vacuum. Radiation hazards are the harmful effects that can occur to the body due to radiations.

Heat and light are forms of radiations that can be felt. Although X-rays are ionizing radiations, they cannot be felt by the skin. Hence, it is important to be aware of radiation hazards and radiation protection.

Natural sources of radiation are radon and cosmic rays. Artificial sources of radiation are: (a) diagnostic radiation in the form of radiography, CT scan, PET scan and nuclear scan; (b) therapeutic radiation in the form of brachytherapy and radiotherapy.

Units of Radiation

As per the International System of Units, dose of ionizing radiation is measured in unit called as gray (Gy). One Gy is defined as that quantity of radiation which results in energy deposition of one Joule per kilogram in the irradiated tissue. Gray has replaced the earlier unit known as the rad. 1 Gy is equal to 100 rads.

Effective dose of radiation is different for different tissues and is measured in terms of a unit called as Sievert (Sv). This depends on the quality factor (Q) of the tissue which permits passage of energy. Dose equivalent (Sv) = Quality factor (Q) × Dose (Gy).

Effects of Radiation

Stochastic effects of radiation are the ones whose probability of occurrence increases with increase in dose and include cancer and genetic effects.

Deterministic effects are the ones which increase in severity with increase in dose and include cataract, blood dyscrasias and impaired fertility.

Irradiation *in utero* can lead to developmental abnormalities (8–25 weeks), cancer which can be expressed in childhood or in adults due to DNA damage by radiation.

Preconception maternal irradiation in therapeutic doses gives rise to defects in 1 out of 10 exposed children. Nonurgent radiological testing should not be done between 8–17 weeks of gestation, which is the most sensitive period for organogenesis.

Children are 10 times more sensitive to hazards of radiations than adults. Hence, radiography with high kV and low mAs technique is recommended in children.

Acute radiation syndrome is said to occur when high doses kill so many cells that tissues and organs are damaged immediately. The higher the radiation dose, the sooner the effects of radiation will appear and higher will be the probability of death. This was seen in atomic bomb survivors in 1945 and emergency workers responding to the 1986 Chernobyl nuclear power plant accident who received radiation to the tune of 800 to 16,000 mSv.

Acute radiation at doses in excess of 100 Gy to the total body, usually result in death within 24 to 48 hrs from neurological and cardiovascular failure. This is known as the cerebrovascular syndrome.

Chronic radiation causes radiation pneumonitis and even permanent scarring that results in respiratory compromise.

AVERAGE EFFECTIVE DOSE IN MILLISIEVERTS (mSv)

X-ray Chest	0.02
CT Orbits	0.8
CT Temporal bone	1.0
CT Head	2.0
CT Spine	3.0
CT Chest	8.0
CT Abdomen	10.0
CT Pelvis	10.0

The International Commission of Radiation Protection (ICRP) was formed in 1928 on the recommendation of the first International Congress of Radiology in 1925 which formed the International Commission on Radiation Units (ICRU). The National Commission for Radiation Protection (NCRP) in America and the Atomic Energy Regulatory Board (AERB) in India are the regulatory bodies that recommend norms for permissible doses of radiation for radiation workers and for the general public.

Atomic Energy Regulatory Board (AERB) which is the Indian Regulatory Board was constituted on November 15, 1983 by the President of India by exercising the powers conferred by Section 27 of the Atomic Energy Act, 1962. The Regulatory Authority of AERB is derived from the rules and notifications promulgated under the Atomic Energy Act, 1962 and the Environmental (Protection) Act, 1986. Radiation safety in handling of radiation generating equipment is governed by Section 17 of the Atomic Energy Act, 1962 and the Radiation Protection Rules, 1971 issued under the Act.

The overall objective of radiation protection is to provide an appropriate standard of protection for man without unduly limiting the beneficial practices giving rise to radiation exposure.

Atomic Energy Regulatory Board (AERB) recommends and lays down guidelines regarding the specifications of medical X-ray equipment, for the room layout of X-ray installation, regarding the work practices in X-ray department, the protective devices and also the responsibilities of the radiation personnel, employer and Radiation Safety Officer (RSO). It is the authority in India which exercises a regulatory control and has the power to decommissioning X-ray installations and also for imposing penalties on any person contravening these rules.

Benefit Risk Analysis

Since radiation exposure entails inherent risks of radiation effects, no decision to expose an individual can be undertaken without weighing benefits of exposure against potential risks, that is, making a benefit risk analysis.

Principles of Radiation Protection

1. Justification of a practice
2. Optimized protection
3. Dose limitation

Radiation Protection Actions

The triad of radiation protection actions comprise of "time-distance-shielding". Reduction of exposure time, increasing distance from source, shielding of patients and occupational workers, have proven to be of great importance.

Shielding

Shielding implies that certain materials (concrete, lead) will attenuate radiation (reduce its intensity) when they are placed between the source of radiation and the exposed individual.

Source Shielding

X-ray tube housing is lined with thin sheets of lead because X-rays produced in the tube are scattered in all directions, to protect both patients and personnel from leakage radiation. AERB recommends a maximum allowable leakage radiation from tube housing not greater than 1 mGy per hour per 100 cm^2.

Structural Shielding

The lead lined walls of radiology department are referred to as protective barriers because they are designed to protect individuals located outside the X-ray rooms from unwanted radiation.

1. Primary barrier is one which is directly struck by the primary or the useful beam.
2. Secondary barrier is one which is exposed to secondary radiation either by leakage from X-ray tube or by scattered radiation from the patient.

The room housing X-ray unit should not be less than 18 m^2 for general purpose radiography and conventional fluoroscopy equipment and that of the CT room housing the gantry of the CT unit should not be less than 25 m^2.

Wall of the X-ray rooms on which primary X-ray beam falls should not be less than 35 cm thick brick or equivalent. Walls of the X-ray room on which scattered X-rays fall should not be less than 23 cm thick brick or equivalent. The walls and viewing window of the control booth should have material of 1.5 mm lead equivalent.

Personnel Shielding

Shielding apparel should be used as and when necessary which comprise of lead aprons, eye glasses with side shields, hand gloves and thyroid shields. The minimum thickness of lead equivalent in the protective apparel should be 0.5 mm. These are classified as a secondary barrier to the effects of ionizing radiation as they protect an individual only from secondary (scattered) radiation and not the primary beam.

Patient Shielding

Thyroid, breast and gonads are shielded to protect these organs especially in children and young adults.

The responsibility for establishing a Radiation Protection Program rests with the hospital administration/owners of the X-ray facility. The administration is expected to appoint a Radiation Safety Committee (RSC) and a Radiation Safety Officer (RSO).

Every radiation worker prior to commencing radiation work and at subsequent intervals not exceeding 12 months shall be subjected to the medical examination. Radiation Safety Officer (RSO) should be an individual with extensive training and education in areas such as radiation protection, radiation physics, radiation biology, instrumentation, dosimetry and shielding design. Duties include assisting the employer in meeting the relevant regulatory requirements applicable to the X-ray installation and ensuring that all radiation measuring and monitoring instruments under custody are properly calibrated and maintained in good condition.

Recommended Dose Limits

Once pregnancy is established the dose equivalent to the surface of pregnant woman's abdomen should not exceed 2 mSv for the remainder of the pregnancy. Ten Day Rule states that all females of reproductive age who need an X-ray examination should get it done within first 10 days of menses to avoid irradiation to possible conception.

As a general principle radiation exposure should be less than 20 mSv/year for radiation workers and less than 1 mSv/year for general public.

Optimization of protection can be achieved by optimizing the procedure to administer a radiation dose which is as low as reasonably achievable (ALARA), so as to derive maximum diagnostic information with minimum discomfort to the patient.

Detection of Radiation

Following methods of detecting radiation, based on physical and chemical effects produced by radiation exposure, are available:

1. *Ionization*: The ability of radiation to produce ionization in air is the basis for radiation detection by the ionization chamber.
2. *Photographic effect*: The ability of radiation to blacken photographic film is the basis of detectors that use film.
3. *Luminescence*: When radiation strikes certain materials they emit light that is proportional to the radiation intensity.

4. *Scintillation*: Here radiation is converted into light, which is then directed to a photomultiplier tube, which then converts the light into an electrical pulse.

Personnel dosimetry is the monitoring of individuals who are exposed to radiation during the course of their work. It is accomplished through the use of devices such as the pocket dosimeter, the film badge or the thermoluminescent dosimeter (TLD). The dose is subsequently stated as an estimate of the effective dose equivalent to the whole body in mSv for the reporting period. Dosimeters used for personnel monitoring have dose measurement limit of 0.1–0.2 mSv (10–20 mrem).

Thermoluminescent dosimeter can measure exposures as low as 1.3 μC/kg (5 mR) and the pocket dosimeter can measure up to 50 μC/kg (200 mR). The film badge however cannot measure exposures < 2.6 μC/kg (10 mR). TLD can withstand certain degree of heat, humidity and pressure, their crystals are reusable and instantaneous readings are possible if the department has a TLD analyzer. The greatest disadvantage of a TLD is its cost.

Index

D

E

N

O

P

R